All author royalties for this book will be donated to The BEEP Fund Ltd

The BEEP Fund Ltd. was set up in 1994 and is a Cumbrian based pre-hospital care charity. BEEP stands for 'Bringing Enhanced Emergency care to Patients'. The charity raises money to pay for the training and supply of medical equipment to a group of doctors who volunteer their time to provide enhanced medical care in the pre-hospital environment, whether that is on the roadside at the scene of a traffic accident or in someone's home during a life-threatening emergency.

All of the Doctors work in other areas of the NHS including Accident and Emergency, Anaesthetics and General Practice. Some of them also work for the local Air Ambulance team (the Great North Air Ambulance). Much of the medical equipment they carry is more sophisticated than what is provided on front line NHS ambulances, including portable ultrasound scanners and surgical equipment. Our team of volunteer BEEP Doctors are on call 24/7 to provide a level of enhanced clinical care in medical emergencies that cannot be provided by even the most highly skilled paramedics, though they do work closely alongside these paramedics. These skills include pre-hospital anaesthetics, surgical procedures and provision of a broader spectrum of drugs, all of which allows for better stabilisation of seriously ill patients long before they reach hospital. This is especially important where the journey times to hospital can be extremely long, such as in the more rural areas of Cumbria. Effectively they are bringing the Accident and Emergency Room to the patient.

Our team of fourteen doctors cover the majority of Cumbria from Workington in the West; Brampton and Alston in the East; Gretna and the Scottish Borders in the North and Kendal and Morecambe in the South. The BEEP Doctors attend the most serious medical incidents in the county, including road traffic collisions, farming accidents or other life-threatening emergencies. They work under the governance of the North West Ambulance Service who are the ones responsible for calling them out to these emergencies. As well as being highly trained and experienced in pre-hospital medical care, they also respond in their own cars using blue lights and sirens, for which they have also had additional training.

More information can be found on their web site: www.beepfund.org.uk

THE
NHS
THE STORY SO FAR

Ellen Welch

PEN & SWORD
HISTORY

AN IMPRINT OF PEN & SWORD BOOKS LTD.
YORKSHIRE - PHILADELPHIA

First published in Great Britain in 2018 under the title
The NHS at 70: A Living History and reprinted in this revised format in 2020 by
PEN AND SWORD HISTORY
an imprint of
Pen & Sword Books Ltd
Yorkshire - Philadelphia

ISBN 978 1 39900 081 9

Typeset in Sabon 11/13.5 By
SJmagic DESIGN SERVICES, India.
Printed and bound in England
by CPI Group (UK) Ltd, Croydon, CR0 4YY.

Pen & Sword Books Ltd incorporates the Imprints of Pen & Sword Books
Archaeology, Atlas, Aviation, Battleground, Discovery, Family History, History,
Maritime, Military, Naval, Politics, Railways, Select, Transport, True Crime,
Fiction, Frontline Books, Leo Cooper, Praetorian Press, Seaforth Publishing,
Wharncliffe and White Owl.

For a complete list of Pen & Sword titles please contact

PEN & SWORD BOOKS LIMITED
47 Church Street, Barnsley, South Yorkshire, S70 2AS, England
E-mail: enquiries@pen-and-sword.co.uk
Website: www.pen-and-sword.co.uk

Contents

Acknowledgements

When I agreed to write a book on the history of the NHS in time for the 70th birthday celebrations, I hadn't really appreciated the scale of the project I had taken on. Writing a second edition to include a chapter on the coronavirus pandemic has felt equally daunting. Encapsulating an institution which has undergone so many changes, and presenting it as something readable, was an overwhelming prospect and since the NHS has been described as the closest thing the English people have to a religion, I felt a weight of responsibility to do it justice. I have a lot of people to thank for helping me finish it.

The personal accounts are what bring this book to life. All of us in the UK have an NHS story to tell, and I would have liked to fill the pages with many more. I am indebted to all of the contributors, who took the time to write their accounts - a massive thank you for your efforts to Noreen and Janyce Quigley, Rose Singleton, Kate Cavanagh, Meg Parkes, Geoff Gill, Judith Susser, David Wingfield, Lianna Brinded, Hannah Ramsdale, Alison Gill, Neil Barnard, Irina Bardsley Carol Trow, Jenny Abthorpe, Rebecca Daly and Denise Tyrell and her family, especially Nevilla and Lauren. Thanks to Karyn Burnham for her editing skills and to the entire team at Pen and Sword for bringing the final product together. Many thanks too to Dr Andrew Stein for his encouragement, comments and contributions to chapter 5.

As a declaration of interests, I am a doctor, and I have worked in both public and private healthcare settings in the UK and New Zealand and as a cruise ship doctor in an American system. The views in this book are my own. I am by no means an 'NHS expert' and in fact I learnt a lot about the NHS during my research for this book. In the further reading section, I point you towards the texts of many more learned people who have spent years writing about the NHS and health policy, and whose work helped to shape this book. I have attempted to transform the history of the NHS into a digestible book that can be understood. All facts and figures are from references sources, which have not been highlighted in the text to make it an easier read, but can be found at the back of the book, and I am happy to have any inaccuracies corrected.

Preface to the Second Edition

The Coronavirus pandemic has changed life as we know it across the world. Here in the UK, the Natonal Health Service has been pushed to centre stage, facing national scrutiny as it responds to an unprecedented crisis.

This book was originally written in 2018, to coincide with the 70th birthday celebrations of the NHS. The second edition has been updated to consider how the NHS has coped with COVID-19. As with any crisis, looking back into history at similar events can help us to learn lessons, and chapter 5 rewinds 100 years to the last worldwide pandemic – the 'Spanish Flu' of 1918.

In the first edition of this book, the 1918 Influenza Pandemic (Spanish Flu) didn't get a look in. I wondered how I could have missed even mentioning the 'greatest massacre' of the twentieth century – its presence changed the world and shaped the health care systems we use today. Spanish Flu infected one in three people on earth and killed up to 100million people. To put this into context, the First World War claimed 17 million lives and the Second World War, 60 million. The history books gloss over the pandemic, mentioning it only as an addendum to the Great War. This can be attributed in part, to attitudes at the time, which considered those who died in battle to be brave and honourable. To die from flu was the opposite of this and made otherwise brave soldiers appear weak. In Germany, it was standard practice for the families of those who died in service to be given a card stating the cause of death. Cards issued for the soldiers who died of flu often failed to mention the disease, stating instead that they died a heroic death for the fatherland.

Laura Spinney, in her book Pale Rider, describes how Spanish flu changed the world by reshaping populations and influencing the course of the First World War. It pushed India towards independance, Switzerland to the brink of civil war and South Africa towards apartheid. Perhaps most relevant to this book – it ushered in universal health care, recognising the need to co-ordinate public health at a national and international level. It changed accepted beliefs that illness was a moral failing and prompted leaders to revamp their health ministries an instigate robust methods of gathering health data.

COVID-19 has also changed the world as we know it. At the time of writing we are far from the end of the pandemic, yet we are in the midst of the deepest recession of the past 150 years. We have confined ourselves to our houses and avoided shops, restaurants, offices and schools for months – will life return to 'normal' when this is all over? Many questions remain unanswered. Will there be a second wave? Will a vaccine control the pandemic? When will it be available, and will it be effective?

The answers to these questions remain uncertain. One thing that is sure, is that the people of the NHS stepped up during this pandemic to care for their communities. As the nation clapped in the streets and declared them heroes, frontline staff quickly adapted to new ways of working to protect the public, often while struggling to protect themselves with inadequate personal protective equiptment. Retired clinicians returned to bolster the workforce and students started work early. Routine work was put on hold to make way for the acute care of large volumes of critically ill patients. GPs transformed their practices overnight to enable consultations to be done primarily over telephone and video.

Most tragically, over 540 health and social care workers in the UK paid the ultimate price and lost their lives to the virus. At the time of writing, this was among the highest number of healthcare worker deaths in the world, second only to Russia. Early studies have indicated that Black, Asian and minority ethnic staff are over represented in these figures. Campaign groups have called for a rigorous public enquiry into the government's response to the pandemic, but this is too little too late for these people, who should have been kept safe as they cared for others.

This book shares some of the stories of the NHS staff who worked through the pandemic, and aims to arm the reader with some knowledge of what the NHS is – where it came from and how it works today so that we can understand the service better to enable us to use it responsibly and have reasonable expectations about what it can provide.

Preface to the First Edition

'Medical treatment should be made available to rich and poor alike in accordance with medical need and no other criteria. The essence of a satisfactory health service is that the rich and poor are treated alike. Poverty is not a disability and wealth is not an advantage.'

Aneurin Bevan – Health Secretary 1946

At midnight on 5th July 1948, the National Health Service was born, with the founding principle to be free at the point of use, and based on clinical need rather than on a person's ability to pay. Seventy years since its formation, these core principles still hold true, although the world we now live in is a very different place to the post-war era in which it was formed, and the long-term sustainability of the service in its current form is questionable.

Broken from two World Wars, undernourished with rationing still in place, and relying on a bucket in front of the fire for the weekly wash – the average life expectancy in 1948 was 60 years old. A child born in 2020 can expect to live to the age of 81.2 years. Over the last century, infant mortality rates have fallen dramatically as standards of living have improved. Immunisation has virtually eliminated death from infectious diseases such as measles, mumps, rubella, poliomyelitis, diphtheria, tetanus and whooping cough. In 1901, the majority of people died young – 75 per cent of deaths were in people under the age of 65 typically from infectious diseases; over a century later, this number is less than 20 per cent. Covid-19 aside, the battle against infectious diseases is largely won and the NHS now faces different challenges, as people are living longer with multiple chronic diseases.

The twentieth century was rife with innovation. The discovery of DNA in the 1950s helped to revolutionise the future prevention and treatment of many diseases. Organ transplants, now a commonplace procedure, were pioneered in the 1960s, and milestones in women's rights and fertility were achieved with the legalisation of abortion and improved accessibility to the contraceptive pill. The 1970s saw the introduction of CT scans, MRI scanners and 'test tube babies; and in the 1980s, cancer treatments improved and breast screening was introduced. We now have expert patients and health charities, and a very different GP waiting room to the one of 1948.

The NHS is the largest and oldest publicly funded healthcare system in the world and provides anyone registered with an NHS number with medical care, without a medical bill at the end of the consultation. It is funded chiefly from taxation and National Insurance contributions. In the early 1950s, charges were introduced for dental services, prescriptions and spectacles (prompting Bevan to resign from cabinet in protest). Today, as we live longer, demand for services continues to grow, and the NHS budget gets stretched thinner and thinner, it has been suggested that people start paying for other NHS services such as routine appointments to see their GP. The slow privatisation of the NHS is moving away from the core values that it was founded upon. Are these values idealistic and unsustainable in modern Britain? Danny Boyle's 2012 Olympic Games opening ceremony brought a tear to many an eye, celebrating the NHS as 'the institution which more than any other unites our nation'. To avoid a move to an American system, where people are bankrupted for medical care, or resort to 'go fund me' pages to raise money to pay for emergency surgery then something does need to change. Less political involvement would help. Health policies need to be evidence based and sustainable, and not formulated to win the next election.

This book attempts to summarise the foundations of the NHS and discuss why it was formed, provide an understanding of its current structure and problems and consider what the future may hold.

Chapter 1

Pre-NHS Britain

Organised health care really started to take shape in the nineteenth century, but clearly medicine and healthcare have been around a whole lot longer than this. Whole libraries are dedicated to the history of medicine, and this chapter aims to present a snapshot of healthcare and medicine over the last few centuries, to gain a flavour of what Britain was like, and to appreciate how life has evolved into the system we know today.

The Middle Ages (500-1500) and The Renaissance (1400-1700)

Medieval medics were pretty powerless in the face of disease, and medical knowledge and ideas about treatments were often based on superstition. The cause of disease was considered supernatural, and herbal remedies were commonplace.

Responsibility for the poor, sick and elderly traditionally fell to the church, and prior to the development of hospitals, townsfolk would turn to their nearest monastery for help with their sick. Prayer rituals were used to heal, and monks produced some of the earliest medical texts documenting the herbal mixtures they used to return their patients back to good health. Religious men were forbidden to spill blood (by Papal decree), so it was common at the time for barbers to assist monks in procedures considered dirty and beneath them – such as bloodletting and leeching, extracting teeth, lancing boils and doing a quick short back and sides (Box 1.1)

Box 1.1 Barber Surgeons

Left: A barber-surgeon extracting stones from a woman's head; symbolising the expulsion of 'folly' (insanity). Watercolour by J. Cats, 1787, after B. Maton. (Wellcome Collection)

Below: High Street of Edinburgh in the 18th century – Note the barber-surgeon's pole with bleeding bowl on the left. Lithograph by W and A K Johnston, 1852 (M McLaren, The Capital Of Scotland, Edinburgh 1950) (via Wikimedia Commons)

For centuries, surgery was a craft carried out by barbers, and early versions of the Hippocratic Oath actually cautioned physicians from practicing surgery. Medieval barbers provided their patients with analgesia using substances such as opium, mandrake root, and hemlock, and, if they didn't pass away due to intoxication, surgery could be performed using wine to clean the wounds. Minor procedures and teeth pulling were commonplace, but internal surgery was also attempted, such as removal of bladder stones, castration of local rapists, and trephining the skulls of epileptic patients to allow the demons to escape. Bloodletting was one of their key duties. It was believed that draining away blood would also drain away the disease. Physicians still considered themselves the 'real doctors' and even when hospitals were established, the barbers did not have a place there, and typically practiced in marketplaces, advertising their business with the familiar red and white striped pole – still seen outside modern hairdressers today – which represented blood and bandages.

As universities developed during the Renaissance, anatomy and surgery began to be studied in more detail. A split formed between academically trained surgeons, who wore long robes, and the 'trained on the job' barber surgeons, who wore shorter robes. In 1540, barbers and surgeons joined forces to gain credibility for their trade and formed the Company of Barber Surgeons. The invention of gunpowder led to new injuries during warfare and barber surgeons such as Frenchman Ambroise Paré made headlines for his work inventing surgical instruments and improving surgical treatments. The advent of anaesthesia and aseptic techniques improved complication and infection rates and as more patients benefited, surgeons gained greater respect. Gradually, due to pressure from the medical profession to distinguish themselves from lesser esteemed back street barbers, surgeons split away from the Company of Barbers to form the Royal College of Surgeons in 1800 and began to hold exams for membership. Prior to this, surgeons were not legally permitted to prescribe internal medicines for their patients – this was a privilege reserved for the learned physicians, who had earned their doctorates of medicine at University. One tradition that still persists to this day is the use of the title 'Mr' or 'Miss' instead of 'Dr' when surgeons qualify as a Member of the Royal College of Surgeons, as a nod to their roots. All surgeons clearly now have to pass a medical degree prior to their years of training in surgery, and they are no longer required to perform haircuts.

In the late 1530s, there were nearly 900 religious houses in England, whose primary function was to provide lodging for travellers and pilgrims, and to act as almshouses and schools. They typically imposed local taxes to assist them in providing such charity. Following the Dissolution of the Monasteries (1536-1540) by Henry VIII, almost all of these institutions were disbanded, creating considerable hardship for the poor and destitute who were thrown out onto the street. Only three London hospitals survived the dissolution, after the citizens of the city petitioned for them to remain – St Barthlolomew's (Bart's), St Thomas's and St Mary's of Bethlehem. They were endowed by the king himself, as the first example of secular support being provided for medical institutions. They remained the principal hospitals in the country until the voluntary hospital movement began in the nineteenth century.

The Renaissance was a period of discovery in medicine. The scientific method was established, and universities established schools of medicine. Artists such as Da Vinci revolutionized painting, and dissection allowed the human body to be studied in more detail, which improved knowledge of anatomy. The invention of the printing press allowed ideas to be disseminated more quickly around Europe, allowing knowledge to be shared. In the 1620s, William Harvey showed that blood circulates, challenging Galen's theory of humours (that disease was due to an imbalance of the four humours – blood, phlegm, black bile and yellow bile) which had been fundamental for centuries; and queried the need for the well-established practice of bloodletting.

Outbreaks of infection still defied medical knowledge. The Black Plague rampaged through Europe in the fourteenth century, recurring in outbreaks until the nineteenth century, claiming over 200 million lives. People believed the pandemic was a punishment from God, and blame was dispensed indiscriminately to groups deemed responsible – such as beggars, lepers, Jews and pilgrims. Individuals with skin diseases such as acne or psoriasis were exterminated, and religious fanaticism bloomed. 'Cures' for the plague included pressing a plucked chicken against the plague sores; smoking tobacco (a novel substance recently introduced from the New World); use of posies and perfumes; dried toad; leeches; a lucky hares foot We now know that plague can be successfully treated with antibiotics, but these, along with public health measures, had not yet been discovered.

Modern History

Improvements in public health and understanding of infection began to develop in the 1800s. In 1796, Edward Jenner discovered vaccinations, by famously using cowpox to protect against smallpox; and some 60 years later, Louis Pasteur developed germ theory, which proved a link between dirt and disease.

The Industrial Revolution resulted in more families moving to towns and cities, often sharing squalid, overcrowded accommodation, and standards of public health were poor. Pollution, contaminated water and a limited diet allowed infectious diseases to flourish and cholera epidemics were common place. An increased understanding of disease and hygiene led to improvements in public health standards. In 1854, John Snow showed the source of the London cholera epidemic to be the communal water pump used at Broad Street. Edwin Chadwick was a social reformer, who worked with the Poor Law Commission. He raised awareness that dirt and squalor are associated with high mortality rates, and that the misery faced by the poor was something the government could control, and not due to some innate shortcoming of the working class. His work led to the first Public Health Act in Britain in 1848, 100 years prior to the creation of the NHS. This led to improvements in the sewage system and building regulations, which contributed to declining mortality rates.

During the nineteenth and early twentieth centuries, great advances were seen in medicine and public health. Anaesthesia and aseptic surgery were introduced; game changing discoveries were made – such as penicillin, x-rays and radium, and blood groups which enabled blood transfusion. The two World Wars shaped medicine. The injuries caused by the heavy artillery of the First World War meant that medicine was forced to pioneer new techniques in plastic surgery and skin grafting, and develop specialities such as maxillofacial surgery. The influenza pandemic of 1918 overshadowed the end of the war, and will be covered in chapter 5. Rationing improved the diets of some and encouraged healthy eating. Events during the Second World War created the stage for the formation of the NHS. Social barriers were broken down and brought people together, looking for improvements in society – more about this in chapter 2.

Workhouses and the Poor Law

The history of the workhouse as an institution to solve the enduring problem of poverty spans over three centuries and was an important

Sampson Kempthorne Workhouse designed for 300 paupers. Sampson Kempthorne (1809–1873) (via Wikimedia Commons)

1. Work Room
2. Store
3. Receiving Wards, 3 beds
4. Bath
5. Washing Room
6. Receiving Ward, 3 beds
7. Washing Room
8. Work Room
9. Flour and Mill Room
10. Coals
11. Bakehouse
12. Bread Room
13. Searching Room
14. Porter's Room
15. Store
16. Potatoes
17. Coals
18. Work Room
19. Washing Room
20. Receiving Ward, 3 beds
21. Washing Room
22. Bath
23. Receiving Ward, 3 beds
24. Laundry
25. Wash-house
26. Dead House
27. Refractory Ward
28. Work Room
29. Piggery
30. Slaughter House
31. Work Room
32. Refractory Ward
33. Dead House
34. Women's Stairs to Dining Hall
35. Men's Stairs to ditto
36. Boys' and Girls' School and Dining Room
37. Delivery
38. Passage
39. Well
40. Cellar under ground

precursor to the NHS. During the reign of Elizabeth I, in 1601, the Act for the Relief of the Poor (which is now known as the Old Poor Law) was passed to deal with beggars, who were viewed as a threat to civil order. This Act made local parishes responsible for the poor and decreed that the 'impotent poor' – the old and sick – were to be cared for in poorhouses, while able bodied paupers should be given work and sent to prison if they refused. Individual parishes were responsible for overseeing their own areas, and at its inception, local populations were small enough for communities to be aware of each other's circumstances, meaning the 'idle poor' were unable to abuse the system. Relief under the 'Old Poor Law' was either in the form of 'indoor relief' – assistance inside a workhouse or almshouse – or 'outdoor relief', which involved payment in the form of money, food, blankets or clothing. Funding to provide this assistance was collected by Overseers of the Poor, who levied local property owners (a tax that we still pay today now, known as council tax).

There was no uniformity to the system throughout the country, and many paupers migrated towards the more generous parishes. During the seventeenth century, the workhouses evolved as a way of allowing parishes to avoid outdoor relief payments. By 1776, in London alone, over 16,000 people were housed in one of the city's eighty workhouses – which amounted to 1-2 per cent per cent of the capital's population. There was rumbling dissatisfaction with this system, and its critics considered the conditions in many of these 'Paupers Palaces' to be too comfortable, encouraging idleness and pauperism. The New Poor Law was therefore passed in 1834, to cut expenditure and abolish pauperism by attempting to ensure only the truly destitute would accept poor relief. Those eligible could not be better off than the worst paid independent worker, and if they were truly needy, they would be offered the workhouse – a harsh and austere regimen which only the desperate would enter willingly. It was not a prison, and people could come and go if they found work, but the regime was strict and to go into the workhouse was considered the ultimate degradation. Poverty was considered to be a moral failing rather than a misfortune. Inmates' heads were shaved and they were given rough, uncomfortable workhouse uniforms to wear. They engaged in manual labour such as stone breaking and rope picking. Food provided was basic and monotonous such as gruel (watery porridge – Oliver Twist style), broth, bread and beer (safer than water). Orphaned children would be housed alongside unmarried mothers, the elderly, and the mentally and physically ill – conditions were overcrowded and dirty.

Families were separated and parents had restricted contact with their children, often only seeing them once a week for a few hours. Many workhouses had designated wards or annexes for sick paupers, and the nursing care was often carried out by other inmates. Paid nursing, during this period, was considered a job for poor, elderly women and was associated with drunkenness, bad language and a casual attitude to patients. Workhouse unions at the time were required to appoint a medical officer, who was usually part time and poorly paid. Joseph Rogers wrote his memoirs about his time as the workhouse doctor at the Strand Union Workhouse. He reported that he had no qualified nurses to care for over 500 sick inmates. If he wished to administer medication, the bill for this would come out of his pay of £50 a year, meaning that treating patients prevented him from making a living. He described workhouse doctors who routinely gave coloured water for every ailment to avoid medication charges.

Standards continued to be poor until concerns were raised in the 1860s. Prominent figures of the day such as Florence Nightingale commented that these hospitals were as bad, or worse than the military hospitals she had encountered during the Crimean War (1853-1856). In 1865 the medical journal *The Lancet* investigated conditions in workhouse infirmaries and produced scathing reports, which prompted the government to conduct their own inquiries. Inspectors found poorly ventilated wards with no washing facilities. They found infectious fever patients scattered through the wards infecting other inmates. 'Lunatics' shared wards with no medical supervision. The only paid nurse employed at the Rotherhithe workhouse infirmary, Matilda Beeton, spoke of her experiences, reporting that untrained pauper nurses beat the patients and stole their food. She reported dirty patients, crawling with vermin and sleeping in maggot infested beds, and 'an insufficiency of everything', complaining that the same towels used for wiping down patients were used as teacloths. 'It did not seem to me,' said Beeton, 'that a pauper's life was regarded in any other light than the sooner they were dead the better.'

By the end of the nineteenth century, parliament passed the Metropolitan Poor Act, to improve these appalling conditions; which authorised the building of separate workhouse infirmaries, with trained medical and nursing staff. Nightingale and her contemporaries helped to change the attitudes of the day, setting up organised training schools and emphasising the need for properly trained nurses in all hospitals.

In addition to these poor law institutes, local authorities (the Metropolitan Asylums Board) set up institutions which could be accessed by the entire population, not just the poor. Hospitals were built specifically to care for fever patients – those suffering from infectious diseases such as smallpox and tuberculosis – and asylums for the mentally ill. This publicly owned system of hospitals was effectively the foundation for what became the NHS in 1948. This process started in 1929, when a further Act of Parliament transferred the powers and responsibilities of the Poor Law to local government authorities, who took over the administration of the poor law infirmaries, as well as the fever hospitals and asylums.

Winter in the Workhouse The *Graphic*, 21 December 1907 (unknown author via Wikimedia Commons)

Florence Nightingale (1820-1910)

Florence Nightingale was a celebrated British nurse and the founder of modern nursing. She became famed as the 'Lady with the Lamp' during the Crimean War, when she took a team of nurses out to improve the conditions and cleanliness in the military hospitals. Nightingale was a believer in the miasma theory, that disease was spread through foul air, and pointed out that more troops died from diseases such as cholera, typhoid and dysentery than from their battle wounds, and she campaigned for improved sanitation. Her nightly rounds with her lamp, checking on the soldiers gained their respect and she returned to Britain a heroine. Donations poured into her 'Nightingale fund' which she used to establish the Nightingale Training School at St Thomas's Hospital in London, which transformed nursing from a lowly, unwholesome job, to a professional career, teaching nurses discipline and practical skills. She pioneered infection control measures and influenced ward designs, realising that the setup of a hospital can affect the health and recovery of its patients, and the classic 'Nightingale wards' as shown on page 22 bear her name.

Florence Nightingale circa 1860. (via Wikimedia Commons)

NO. 9 WARD, ROYAL INFIRMARY, LIVERPOOL, May 1911

Nightingale ward 1911– Royal Liverpool Infirmary (Used with permission from The Liverpool Nurses League)

Voluntary Hospitals

In stark contrast to these municipal or public hospitals were the Voluntary hospitals. 'Voluntaries' as they were known, were funded by the voluntary contributions of investors and philanthropists. Many had been founded centuries before and they included most of London's best-known teaching hospitals and some smaller cottage hospitals run by GPs in more rural areas. Some, like Bart's, claimed a medieval origin, while many more were formed in the early eighteenth century, such as the Edinburgh Royal Infirmary, the Bristol Royal Infirmary and Addenbrookes in Cambridge. Voluntary hospitals were autonomous and could choose not only who they wanted to employ, but who they wanted to treat. Charitable donations were dependent on high cure rates, meaning that elderly patients and those with chronic disease were unlikely to be admitted. The voluntary hospitals were renowned for cutting edge medicine and medical education; and in 1834, the Select Committee on Medical Education commented that these voluntary hospitals were a major source of the advancement

22

of medical science. The voluntary hospitals had strict admission criteria, requiring either a letter of recommendation from a hospital governor or subscriber, or the payment of fees. The payment of fees was variable – some were paid by family and friends or by the parish; while others prepared for being sick, by making weekly payments to a hospital contributory scheme. All patients were required to provide financial security to cover burial costs if they died in hospital. In some cases, hospitals would waive fees, in cases of extreme need. Many hospitals would reject patients suffering with venereal disease, and hospitals such as St Thomas's, that did accept them, housed them in designated 'foul wards' and upped their fees (10s 6d versus 3s 6d in the late eighteenth century). Hospital patients tended to come from the lower classes, as the wealthy preferred to pay doctors to treat them in their own homes.

In the 1890s, the voluntary hospitals ran alongside the local government and poor law hospitals, providing approximately 26 per cent per cent of the nation's beds, leaving the majority of the chronically unwell and psychiatric cases to the other institutes. This figure rose to 33 per cent per cent in 1938. As medicine advanced and there was a focus on teaching and research, doctors (and governors) in voluntary hospitals became even more selective of their patients; choosing those with diseases of interest, or of a short term nature to ensure a rapid turnover of patients. This rigid system led the way for the expansion of the old workhouse or public hospitals to fill the gaps. By the 1920s, many of these 'workhouse infirmaries' were larger than the old workhouses themselves. Many had resident medical staff and facilities for x-rays, laboratory tests and surgery. It became customary for the voluntaries to transfer their 'unwanted cases' such as cancer patients, or those with infectious disease, to the local authority hospitals.

Through the 1930s and 1940s, pressure for reform of health services grew. Charity donations, which the voluntaries depended on, declined, and the emergency response coordinated by the government during wartime – which involved all the hospitals working together to share staff and resources – demonstrated how a universal system may work. Bevan's NHS Act's brought the voluntary hospitals into public ownership, and from then on, they were funded from general taxation, staffed by salaried consultants and professional administrators.

My NHS Story

Noreen Quigley is a retired nurse from County Durham who completed her training at the dawn of the NHS. (Oral history taken by her daughter Janyce Quigley)

'I started my nurse training aged 17 as a "pre-probationer" in 1946 at Holmside and South Moor Hospital, which was a cottage hospital with about 48 beds for miners and their families. When I was 18, I moved to Sunderland General Hospital where I trained as a State Registered Nurse (SRN) for 3 years and in those days, you lived at the hospital where you trained. You had to be back in the nurse's home, signed in on a register by 10pm at night – I won't tell you the number of times I slipped down the fire escape to go to a dance! As soon as I finished, I received a letter from the Matron back at the miner's hospital offering

Noreen Quigley, 1950.

me a position as night sister and I was amazed to be told I could live at home. I returned there when I was 21, in 1950, and it was no longer a miner's hospital, but an NHS hospital.

'I loved being a nurse. You really had to want to do the job back then, as the times were difficult, and it was hard physical work, but I liked it a lot. Nursing seems different now, and when I visit hospitals, all I seem to see is nurses writing. I was a night sister for general surgery and medicine. We worked 12-hour shifts starting at 20:15 until 0815 the following day. We checked pressure points twice a day. Matron did her rounds every morning, and woe betide us if she found even a speck of dust during her inspections. We had side wards for the sickest patients, but these were also used for private patients. We looked after them the same as the NHS patients, but the surgeon would be the one who benefited. I never agreed with having private patients in an NHS hospital.'

Late for Duty
(Liverpool Nurses League)

The Dispensaries

Dispensaries formed a key part of healthcare for several hundred years, before they were absorbed into the NHS in 1948, and then largely forgotten. They were charitable organisations, where medical advice and medications could be dispensed – generally for free, or for a minimal fee, and if patients could afford to pay for a doctor, then they were not supposed to make use of the dispensaries. They ran on a subscriber system, similar to that used in the Voluntary hospitals, which relied on the funding of rich philanthropists; this would select patients from the 'deserving poor' to use the services they had sponsored. They would introduce the patient to the dispensary by handing over a note. These institutes were economical in comparison to the hospitals and provided a service somewhere in between the workhouse and the Voluntary hospital. Doctors worked for free, which contributed to their prestige and may have increased their income from private patients. Dispensaries also provided a valuable training experience for doctors, who often dealt with people whose illnesses would not be allowed into the voluntary hospitals – such as infectious cases, or hopeless cases where patients were too ill to leave their homes. In housebound cases, dispensary doctors would visit to diagnose and treat the patient, but only if they lived within 'the dispensary area' and could produce a note from a subscriber. If they could not, then they would be passed over to the care of the poor law – which generally meant admission to a workhouse. The NHS removed the need for the dispensaries, however volunteers do still play a role in modern health care today, with over 3 million people volunteering in acute trusts, taking on roles such as befriending, hospitality, entertainment and administrative support.

General Practice

Prior to the twentieth century, general practitioners worked privately, treating people who had the means to pay, often in their own homes. In 1911, the Chancellor of the Exchequer, Lloyd George, introduced the National Insurance Act, which was very influential in the development of primary care. It aimed to relieve hardship among the working classes during periods of illness, and made health insurance compulsory for workers, contracting GPs to provide medical services for working people – but not for their families, who were still required to pay.

The Act meant that unemployed workers no longer had to turn to the stigmatised welfare provisions of the Poor Law. All workers who earned less than £160 a year paid 4 pence into the scheme, their employer paid 3 pence and general taxation paid 2 pence – 'ninepence for fourpence'. Workers were then entitled to take sick leave at 10 shillings a week for the first 13 weeks and 5 shillings a week for the next 13. They were given access to free treatment for tuberculosis, and treatment from a panel doctor (or GP) of their choosing when sick. The 'panel' was the term for the list of patients a GP cared for. GPs received an annual capitation fee for patient's on their list (a funding mechanism that still exists today)

A sizeable portion of society were still required to pay for medical treatment, and hospital inpatient care was still not provided to insured workers, meaning that many people continued to experience considerable hardship, until the NHS was established. Many GPs were acutely aware of the unfairness of these financial issues. Dr Andrew Stein is a Consultant in Renal Medicine in Coventry. He recalls the experiences of his father, Dr Maurice Stein, who worked as a pre-NHS GP. An Irish Jew, who served in the RAF throughout the Second World War, he settled in a poor small town in Kent. 'It was hard for Jewish GPs (especially an Irish one) to find enough patients on a panel in the more affluent areas before 1948 - there were ways in which the Establishment blocked them. Instead, they gravitated towards smaller, less popular towns. Many GPs would treat the family of a patient on their panel/list for free. Similarly, for someone really poor with no link to the panel, treatment would go ahead in exchange for payment in kind - such as food or some DIY work. I remember my father working from the front room in our house and patients giving him fresh eggs as a thank you."

My NHS Story

Dr Rose Singleton is a GP working in rural Cumbria, who reflects on her experiences of being a new GP in the NHS:

'In 1924, Dr. Andrew Manson, protagonist of AJ Cronin's novel *The Citadel**, arrived in South Wales to start the first job of his medical career as an assistant to a local GP, Dr Page. He was 24 years old, fresh from medical school in Edinburgh and eager to get started. His growing unease is described in the initial paragraphs, as it becomes clear that Dr Page is incapacitated by a 'far from recent' stroke, and since the departure of the previous assistant, his clinics have been run

---

* The Citadel by AJ Cronin was ground-breaking when published in 1937 dealing with medical ethics and extolling the virtues of socialized medicine. It has been credited with laying the foundations for the formation of the NHS.

by his dispenser. As a new doctor, Andrew is thrust into taking on responsibilities far beyond his comfort zone and without a safety net if things go wrong. Although Andrew Manson is a fictional character, Cronin was a doctor qualifying in 1919, and the novel draws on some of his experiences working in a South Wales mining town in the early twentieth century.

'I qualified 90 years after Cronin and was a junior doctor for seven years before achieving my CCT (certificate of completion of training), allowing me to work independently as a General Practitioner. Post-graduate training of doctors within the NHS is now much better organised, and General Practice is recognised as a specialty in its own right. What happened to Andrew Manson simply wouldn't happen now, with doctors – and of course their patients – being much better off for it.

'Despite this passing of time and the vast improvements in training since 1924, some things don't change; Andrew describes the first patient he sees in his new role, "conscious of his nervousness, his inexperience, his complete unpreparedness for such a task". Away from the bustling wards he felt isolated and under-confident and suddenly had the pressure of making a diagnosis and devising a treatment plan alone. There can't be a doctor who hasn't felt this way, and with each step up in role, from foundation doctor to Registrar, to GP or Consultant, the pressure intensifies and the same uncomfortable feelings come flooding back. The hardest jump to make for me was from GP Registrar to fully qualified GP. After seven years of having my work scrutinised, assessed, and ultimately supervised, I fledged as a GP in the autumn of 2016, tumbling from the safety of my training programme, headlong into independence, and without anyone watching my back. I was reading "H is for Hawk" by Helen Macdonald around that time and I found some unexpected parallels with my experience of starting out in "real" general practice. Her description of becoming an expert, albeit in the art of falconry, really helped me understand why it was so hard: "Being a novice is safe. When you are learning how to do something, you do not have to worry about whether or not you are good at it. But when you have done something, have learned how to do it, you are not safe anymore. Being an expert opens you up to judgement." Although I was always responsible for the decisions I made as a junior doctor, everything I did was under the umbrella of a supervising GP or Consultant and losing that cover upon gaining my CCT was acutely exposing. Any bad decisions, oversights, or mistakes I made from that point forwards would be judged in the context of an expert, a GP, and I could no longer rely on the safety of the novice.

'I remember my first patient as a new GP, it was a toddler with fever. Having worked in paediatrics and through training in general practice, this was a familiar presentation, but by acquiring the title of GP and without the comfort blanket of my trainer to bail me out if I lost confidence, it felt like I was right back at the start, exactly like Andrew Manson. I now also had a permanent job for the first time in my career, I wouldn't just move on after six months, my name appears on hospital letters and patient records and I am cherished by some patients as *their* GP. It was likely I would see the little girl and her family again (and indeed I have done), and I couldn't hide behind a cloak of anonymity, previously granted by rotational junior doctor jobs.

'Being a GP in a small town, and furthermore within the community where I live, has opened my eyes to a network of connections that link people and experiences inextricably to their illness and their wellness. I understand why a lady with terrible osteoarthritis won't accept a hip replacement when I meet her confused old dad, who can't manage without her. The teenager with panic attacks doesn't have to tell me she's worried about cancer, because I know that her school friend recently died from it. I'm starting to see things differently, to see beyond symptoms and diseases, to glimpse the human condition in a way I haven't understood it before. I'm not a medical student anymore, I don't need a proforma for history taking, I'm not a GP trainee, having to follow a defined pattern for communicating with patients, I've developed a relationship with my community, which allows me to understand them in ways that I could barely touch upon as trainee. The breadth of knowledge, understanding and experience is an incredible revelation, but of course it can also be devastating. Imagine a middle-aged lady who comes for advice, wondering why she is struggling to count out the change in her shop. I can smell cigarettes on her breath and notice her clubbed fingers. I can guess without needing tests that she probably has lung cancer with brain metastases. I can see the future; the terrible conversation with her and her family when I tell them the result of the chest x-ray, her agonising realisation that it can't be treated, her death. As her GP, I'll be there through all of it; liaising with her specialists, arranging her palliative care, writing her death certificate and comforting her family when it's all over.

'I continue to find general practice challenging, but incredibly rewarding. There are few jobs, even within medicine, where you can potentially make someone feel better every ten minutes. A good GP can't be replaced by a robot or an app and whilst easy access to good medical advice is important, the role of a GP is so much more than technical nous, the value of which was superbly described by the great medical educationalist William Osler, 'It is much more important to know what sort of a patient has a disease than what sort of a disease a patient has.' The future of the NHS will include gene therapy, robotic surgery and digital health, but someone still has to be there when technology can't be, and I hope that GPs will continue to provide the holistic cornerstone that the NHS so vitally needs, now, and for generations to come.'

Chapter 2

The Formation of the NHS

The NHS was born on 5th July 1948. Doctors, nurses, dentists, opticians, pharmacists and hospitals came together for the first time as one colossal UK organisation, and the unveiling of a hugely ambitious plan to provide free healthcare for all. Aneurin 'Nye' Bevan, the health secretary recognised as its creator, formally launched the service at Trafford General Hospital (known at the time as Park Hospital) in Manchester. The first NHS patient to be treated was 13-year old Sylvia

Aneurin Bevan, Minister of Health, on the first day of the National Health Service, 5 July 1948, at Park Hospital, Davyhulme, near Manchester. (via Wikimedia Commons)

Diggory, who recalls shaking Bevan's hand, saying, 'Mr Bevan asked me if I understood the significance of the occasion and told me that it was a milestone in history – the most civilised step any country had ever taken, and a day I would remember for the rest of my life – and of course, he was right.'

Aneurin Bevan

Aneurin Bevan, or Nye, as he was known, was born in a South Wales mining community in 1897. Growing up, he was exposed to poverty and disease, and three of his nine siblings died during childhood. His father was a coal miner, and Bevan followed in his footsteps, leaving school at age thirteen to work in the local colliery. His involvement in politics started as a miner, when he emerged as one of the leaders in the 1926 Miners' strike, and he was subsequently elected as a Labour MP. Bevan became well known as a champion for the working class, and he made an impression in parliament with his passionate debating style. Following

Labour's landslide victory in 1945, he was appointed Minister for Health by Prime Minister Clement Atlee, and given the task of implementing the manifesto plans for a welfare state and healthcare revolution. Bevan recognised that health was a key factor in social inequalities and made it his mission to tackle this head on.

Aneurin Bevan.
(Geoff Charles via
Wikimedia Commons)

Early twentieth century

The NHS was formed from an amalgamation of the healthcare services that already existed, which at the start of the twentieth century was fragmented and lacked structure and coordination. During this time, most doctors either worked for themselves, or were funded by charitable institutions, and much of the population had no access to their services at all. The state had slowly taken on responsibility for the health of the nation since the Poor Law reforms were implemented in Victorian Britain, leading to improved public health measures: vaccination was made compulsory for children in 1853, and the importance of disease surveillance was recognised.

The dawn of the twentieth century welcomed a Liberal government into power, who tried to reduce poverty and improve people's health by introducing reforms such as school medical inspections and free school meals. They introduced state-funded pensions, mother and baby welfare clinics and set up the health visitor system. Lloyd George's National Health Insurance scheme provided basic medical

Ministry of health 1930. (Wellcome Collection)

care to working men who paid their compulsory contributions to the scheme, which provided the assurance of medical care should they become sick, along with a limited income during periods of unemployment. Many men resented giving up their hard-earned wages to such a scheme, and there were glaring deficiencies to this system – namely, a lack of access to hospital care, and no universal cover for wives and children, who often continued to pay into private health insurance schemes.

In the early twentieth century, it was commonplace for the privileged elite in society to look down on the working classes and the poor, whose supposed inferiority and natural degeneracy were thought to predispose them to disease. Public health policies of the time were influenced by these attitudes, and rather than searching for the cause of illness in the abject living conditions of the lower classes, eugenicists argued that it was their own fault for falling ill, as they lacked the drive to achieve a better quality of life.

The 1918 Influenza Pandemic radically changed this thinking. The disease caused a tidal wave of death, killing an estimated 50-100 million people around the world, showing no discrimination between rich and poor and lasted over two years. (see chapter 5 for more about the pandemic) Health authorities realised that it was no longer reasonable to blame individuals for catching an infectious disease, and that the response to containing a pandemic needed coordination on a population level. The Ministry of Health was established in the midst of the pandemic in 1919, strengthening the philosophy that healthcare is the inherent responsibility of the state. The Ministry took control of the administration of the Poor Law, National Insurance, local government, planning, housing and environmental health. The 1920s saw many governments around the world embracing socialised medicine. Russia was the first country to set up a centralised public healthcare system, funded by a state-run insurance scheme. Germany, France, and eventually the UK followed suit.

Lord Dawson's Report

In 1919, Sir Bertrand Dawson, a military doctor and physician at the London Hospital, was commissioned by the newly formed Ministry of Health to chair a council to advise on the systemised provision of health services to link the hospitals into a single system. His 1920 report outlined a model that would be adopted by the NHS 30 years later, based on primary healthcare centres (staffed by general practitioners) and secondary health centres (hospitals staffed by consultant specialists). The committee's proposal was backed by a report eight years later from the Royal Commission on National Health Insurance who advocated for medical services to be divorced entirely from the insurance system in the same way as public health services – and funded by the general public's purse. The years following this saw a period of depression and economic cuts, which destroyed any chance of significant reform.

The State of Healthcare

By the 1930s, many of the voluntary hospitals faced closure due to financial crises and many were pleading for state support. The charitable donations on which they depended reduced significantly over the years – in the 1890s, 88 per cent per cent of their income came from gifting, and this had dropped to a mere 35 per cent per cent by the 1930s, and many could not keep up with the costs of medical treatment. Furthermore, a national survey of hospitals was conducted in 1938 which indicated that the whole country needed an upgrade. The major problems identified were a shortage of beds due to poor hospital buildings, a shortage of consultants, and poor patient access to both. Lack of a structured system meant that the distribution of specialists around the country was haphazard. Complicated cases were cared for in hospitals without the necessary resources, and those hospitals that could deal with such cases had beds full of more simple cases. Long stay wards were lacking, some reported to have a ratio of 60 patients to 1 trained nurse, accommodating a mix of elderly patients with dementia on the same ward as young children. Furthermore, the cost of being sick was beyond the reach of the average person. A patient diagnosed with tuberculosis, undergoing operative treatment and several months bedrest would be expected to pay more than £1000.

The British Medical Association had proposed in 1930 that health insurance coverage should be given to the whole population, and that a co-ordinated regional hospital service should be instituted. The Socialist Medical Association went a step further and proposed that healthcare should be provided to all, free at the point of use, through a government led scheme. This policy for a state medical service was adopted by the Labour Party at their 1934 conference.

Wartime Healthcare

The threat of another war halted parliamentary discussions on the future of the health service and the Ministry turned their attention to co-ordinating all hospitals to join together to form an Emergency Medical Service (EMS) in preparation for the mass casualties of war. The number of beds in some hospitals was increased and temporary buildings were erected. Many of the former Poor Law institutions were upgraded, and many specialist centres (such as plastic surgery, neurosurgery and rehabilitation units) were created in preparation for war. The Ministry dictated what the functions of the existing hospital should be on a regional basis – which laid the foundation for a united health service when the war was over.

After an air raid. (Reproduced with permission from the British Red Cross Museum and Archives)

Piccadilly underground during the Blitz. (Reproduced with permission from the British Red Cross Museum and Archives)

Voluntary Aid Detachment

During the First World War, the British Red Cross set up the Voluntary Aid Detachment Scheme, and recruited thousands of women volunteers to serve their country providing nursing care. These civilian nurses sought employment in hospitals after the war, ultimately leading to the Registration of Nurses Act in 1919, which only allowed nurses with at least three years formal training to be admitted onto the nursing register.

(Liverpool Nurses League)

The war changed attitudes. The state had controlled most aspects of people's lives during the war – with good effects. Rationing improved the health of the poor, and the EMS response to treating the casualties of air raids had given citizens access to healthcare that they had never experienced before – so the prospect of the government looking after healthcare did not seem outlandish. The major political parties largely agreed on the country's main priorities and generally cooperated to achieve them – namely post-war recovery and the welfare of the people – and the first twinklings of the NHS.

The Beveridge Report

The Beveridge Report of 1942 set out plans for the future of post-war Britain and paved the way for the modern welfare state. Senior civil servant Sir William Beveridge chaired the committee tasked with reviewing social insurance schemes, and the resulting work 'Report on Social Insurance and Allied Services' became more succinctly known as the Beveridge Report. It put forward a scheme of ideas to tackle what he described as the 'five giant evils' that blighted the lives of British people: want; disease; ignorance; squalor and idleness. It advocated a compulsory social security scheme that would provide benefits without means testing. It proposed that all working people should pay a contribution to a state fund that could be used for a comprehensive health service, the avoidance of mass unemployment and a system of children's allowances. The report had piqued media curiosity and was published for public consumption, selling over 600,000 copies.

The white paper 'A National Health Service' was published in 1944 outlining the wartime coalition government's vision for a free, unified health service. It proposed central government management, with responsibility for its provision lying with the Minister for Health. The minister appointed to this position was Aneurin Bevan, whose proposals for the service went further than what had been discussed before, making him the almost single-handed architect of the NHS. In keeping with Labour's commitment to a programme of public ownership, he wanted nationalisation of municipal and voluntary hospitals with funding to come primarily from taxation rather than National Insurance. This regional hospital scheme to replace the local authority boundaries was a shrewd plan, as it meant the control of the hospitals would no longer be so insular, and executive control of all the hospitals would allow for service planning. In 1946, the National Health Service Act (also known as the 'Bevan Act' due to the Minister's influence) received Royal assent.

Structure of the New NHS

The NHS was planned as a three-tier service, with the Minister of Health overseeing it at the top, and three tiers which could interact with each other to suit the needs of the patient to include:

- Hospitals – Both the municipal and voluntary hospitals were nationalised and organised into 14 regional groups, or hospital boards.
- Primary Care – GPs, dentists, pharmacists and opticians all remained as self-employed professionals, contracted (by local executive councils) to provide services to the NHS so that the patient did not have to pay directly.
- Local Authority services – Community services (such as the provision of midwifery and health visiting services, school medical services, ambulance services, immunisation and public health) remained the responsibility of the local authorities.

The Public Health Laboratory Service (PHLS) became part of the NHS in 1948, providing microbiological investigation of outbreaks of infectious disease. It was set up during the Second World War as the Emergency PHLS due to fears around biological warfare. In 1977, the Communicable Disease Surveillane Centre was established within the PHLS to provide national surveillance of disease. In 2003, the PHLS was replaced by the Health Protection Agency, which later became Public Health England in 2013.

Unhappy Doctors

Hospitals in 1948 were in a poor condition following war time bombing. Most had been built in the late 1800s and were beginning to crumble even before the Blitz. As previously mentioned, there was no sort of health system at the time and hospitals had been established over the years in a haphazard fashion. Most relied on GPs and unpaid consultants, who worked for free in exchange for a secure base for private practice.

The relationship between the medical profession and the state has always been guarded. Many doctors were opposed to the establishment of the NHS as they disliked the idea of becoming employees of the state, and the BMA led a vigorous campaign against it, some even comparing Bevan's proposals to Nazi Germany. Hospital doctors relied on private patients to boost their income and were wary of a new system that would endanger this. Bevan was famously reported as 'stuffing their mouths with gold' by allowing consultants to work within the NHS on a salaried basis (plus merit awards) but able to continue to do some lucrative private work within NHS hospitals. Proposals to make GPs salaried were declined and instead they reached a compromise in which they worked for the NHS as contractors and were paid on a capitation basis, based on the number of patients they had on their list, similar in many ways to the old 'panel system'.

The Birth of the NHS

In mid-summer 1948, medical care in the UK became free, for all people including foreigners living temporarily in Britain. Overnight, Bevan was in charge of 2688 hospitals in the UK, describing the new NHS as 'the most civilised step any country has ever taken'. In spite of the bickering, almost everyone was prepared to make the NHS work. 'The war made us realise that we were all neighbours'.

Additional resources for the new NHS were negligible. The same number of doctors and nurses went to work in the same hospitals on 5 July in the same way they had the day before, but what had changed was improved accessibility for patients and a more equitable distribution of existing services. *The Times* commented that the masses had joined the middle classes.

Demand for the NHS exceeded all predictions. During planning, the predicted annual cost was £170million. In its first full year of operation, costs exceeded £305 million. £1 million was budgeted for opticians, but within a year 5.25 million spectacle prescriptions had produced a bill amounting to £32 million. Similarly with prescriptions – in 1947, doctors issued 7 million prescriptions each month, which rose to 19 million per month by 1951.

Commentators in the BMJ in 1949 predicted the rate of NHS expenditure would lead to national ruin. They reasoned that the predicted NHS budgets planned for before its initiation had ignored

YOUR NEW NATIONAL HEALTH SERVICE

On 5th July the new National Health Service starts

Anyone can use it—men, women and children. There are no age limits, and no fees to pay. You can use any part of it, or all of it, as you wish. Your right to use the National Health Service does not depend upon any weekly payments (the National Insurance contributions are mainly for cash benefits such as pensions, unemployment and sick pay).

CHOOSE YOUR DOCTOR NOW

The first thing is to link up with a doctor. When you have done this, your doctor can put you in touch with all other parts of the Scheme as you need them. Your relations with him will be as now, *personal and confidential*. The big difference is that the doctor will not charge you fees. He will be paid, out of public funds to which all contribute as taxpayers.

So *choose your doctor now*. If one doctor cannot accept you, ask another, or ask to be put in touch with one by the new "Executive Council" which has been set up in your area (you can get its address from the Post Office).

If you are already on a doctor's list under the old National Health Insurance Scheme, and do not want to change your doctor, you need *do nothing*. Your name will stay on his list under the new Scheme.

But make arrangements for *your family* now. Get an application form E.C.1 for *each* member of the family either from the doctor you choose, or from any Post Office, Executive Council Office, or Public Library; complete them and give them to the doctor.

There is a lot of work still to be done to get the Service ready. If *you* make *your* arrangements in good time, you will be helping both yourself and your doctor.

Issued by the Department of Health for Scotland

A

This advertisement appears in selected Sunday, Morning and Evening newspapers in Scotland.

National Health Service leaflet May 1948. (via Wikimedia commons) the effects of the aging population and the figures were based on a false conception of health – meaning that before the NHS, people were cured of simpler and cheaper diseases but fell victim to more complex and more expensive diseases – for which the NHS was now footing the bill.

In 1950, Prime Minister Clement Atlee promoted Hugh Gaitskell to be Chancellor of the Exchequer. To balance the budget, he proposed savings of £13 million annually by imposing charges for dentures and spectacles provided by the NHS. Both Nye Bevan and Harold Wilson resigned from government the very next day in protest. The Conservative government went on to introduce charges for prescriptions of one shilling in 1952.

Apart from a period between 1965 and 1968, prescription charges in England have continued ever since. Today, prescriptions cost £9.10 per item and in 2018/19 £576 million revenue was raised for the NHS in England through prescription charges. A system of exemptions[*] for prescription charges is in place, including those on low incomes, pensioners and students, pregnant women and people with long term medical conditions; meaning than on average 90 per cent per cent of all NHS prescriptions are dispensed free of charge. There are growing concerns about wastage of medications prescribed for free, which in 2009 was estimated in the region of £150million of avoidable waste. In March 2020, as COVID-19 took hold, the Prescription Charges Coalition asked for all charges to be suspended throughout the pandemic. This was declined by Health Secretary Matt Hancock, who said that those who are least able to pay already get free prescriptions.

General Practitioners

Before 1948, GPs worked as independent traders treating people who had the money to pay them, often from a consulting room in their own home. In 1911, GPs were contracted by local insurance committees administering Lloyd George's National Insurance Scheme, to provide general medical services, and were paid a capitation fee for every patient registered with them. At the inception of the NHS, this

---

[*] You can find out more about who is eligible for prescription exemptions here: https://www.nhs.uk/using-the-nhs/help-with-health-costs/get-help-with-pre-scription-costs/

independent contractor status was clung to, from a fear of becoming a salaried employee of the state, but this independence was deceptive. GPs continued to be free to organise their own practices, but the work they did for the NHS was controlled by a tightly defined contract. They received a capitation fee for each patient registered with them, and their expenses were averaged and included in this payment-per-patient. No money could pass between patient and doctor (with few exceptions such as payment for a private medical certificate). The NHS Act of 1946 had planned for health centres to be a main feature of primary care. They envisaged clinics aimed at health promotion made up of GPs, dentists and local health authority clinics, funded by the public purse – but this programme was aborted before it even started. Prior to the NHS, a few GPs had made a handsome living by treating wealthy private patients, but the majority were poorly paid, so the NHS provided them with security.

Lord Beveridge had predicted that the initial jump in demand for GPs' services would eventually fall once people became accustomed to the system, but this never happened, and GPs were overwhelmed with demands from patients who had previously avoided seeking care for financial reasons. Within a month, 90 per cent per cent of the population had registered with a GP. Each GP was personally responsible for the care of their patients 24 hours a day, 7 days a week, 365 days a year, meaning single handed doctors could be on call around the clock with no respite. GPs were assigned as the gatekeepers for the NHS, transferring the decision to go for hospital treatment from the patient to the doctor. A patient's guide produced by the Ministry of Health in 1948 declared that the GP would 'arrange for the patient every kind of specialist care he is himself unable to give. Except in emergency, hospital and specialists would not normally accept a patient for advice or treatment unless he has been sent by his family doctor'. This suited hospital consultants, who felt protected from 'trivial' cases. The government enjoyed increased cost effectiveness, while the GPs enjoyed the continuing responsibility for 'their' patients. This changed the relationship between GPs and consultants, who had previously relied on GP referral as a source of private income. Now they had plenty of NHS patients to keep them busy, few consultants made a substantial income privately and no longer had financial reasons to be grateful to GPs. Today, NHS GPs may be run as private businesses, but they differ from private GP practices in that they do not compete for patients or for profit. They work to NHS contracts, follow NHS guidelines, and see NHS patients.

Optometry

Ophthalmic services did not quite fit into the NHS plan. In 1948, most opticians based their business on the provision of spectacles. Many also provided sight tests, but at this time, there was a proportion of the medical profession who opposed the right of ophthalmic opticians to conduct eye examinations. Once the NHS introduced free eye testing there simply was not enough ophthalmologists in the country to meet the demand and opticians gladly took on this role. This eventually led to the profession being recognised with legislation in 1958 to regulate optical professionals in a similar way to doctors and dentists.

Mass produced spectacles were available in the UK in the 1950s and 1960s through the National Health Service. These frames are a typical example. The coil springs secured the frames when the arms hooked behind the ears. (Science Museum, London. Wellcome Images)

After 1948, an influx of patients attended for their free sight testing – many people demanding free spectacles, even when their vision was found to be perfect. By the end of the 1940s, waiting lists of 18 months for spectacles were common, meaning by the time some received their devices, their vision had changed, and they had to return for an updated prescription. By 1950, this was costing the NHS £22 million annually, and in 1951, the end of free spectacles was one of the first cuts to be made in the NHS. The above image shows a typical pair of NHS glasses, which were almost universally loathed by the wearers due to the stigma attached to wearing state subsidised spectacles.

NHS spectacles showed little imagination in terms of design flair. They were made cheaply for robust use and utility rather than fashion.

History of Dentistry in the UK

Rewinding back a few hundred years, the introduction of sugar brought with it a rise in tooth decay and gum disease. Sugar was initially a luxury reserved only for the rich, some even brushed their teeth with honey and sugar paste, and indeed, Queen Elizabeth I was rumoured to have blackened teeth and foul breath. Consumption increased in the general population throughout the eighteenth century as people developed a taste for toffees, fudge and jams – creating a demand for dental care. During this period, they had several options for their toothache. They could turn to the local blacksmith, who was always happy to pull a tooth, they had the barbers and barber surgeons and they also had the travelling tooth drawers. The tooth drawers are considered to be the forefathers of modern dentistry, since they made a living solely from treating teeth. They travelled the country, attracting trade by putting on a show in the market square, dressing as jesters and wearing necklaces of teeth, then they would extract the teeth of willing participants for a fee in full view of the assembled villagers. The role of these 'operators of the teeth' grew to not only removing teeth, but making artificial teeth, and early methods used a carved hippopotamus ivory base, with human teeth riveted in. The source of the human teeth was dubious – they were notably taken from the mouths of dead soldiers from battlefields such as Waterloo, but as demand grew, they were acquired from dissecting rooms, mortuaries and even graveyards. Dentures were extremely expensive and reserved for the higher echelons of society. By the nineteenth century, dentistry had become a respected profession, and in attempts to distinguish medically trained dentists from with quacks such as jewellers who often gave it a go as a lucrative side line, the Royal College of Surgeons instituted a qualification in dentistry, which led to regulation in the same way as doctors.

The importance of good oral hygiene gained attention at the start of the twentieth century. During recruitment for the British army for the Boer War, general poor health had been highlighted, but dental hygiene especially was noted to be dire. From a force of over 200,000 soldiers, there were nearly 7000 admissions to hospital due to dental causes. Strong teeth were essential to tear the rifle paper needed to load a musket, leading to the expression 'You can't fight if you can't bite!' During the First World War, soldiers were issued with toothbrushes – but had allegedly used them to clean their boots instead. The importance of dental care for the troops was recognised which eventually led to the formation of the Army Dental Corps in 1921. The facial trauma seen during the World Wars led to the establishment of specialist oral surgery units. Access to dental care for civilians was lacking and most people avoided a visit until pain forced them into the dentist's chair. When plans were being formed for the NHS, the Friendly and Approved Societies set up under the 1911 National Insurance Act shared their figures, which showed that in the 1930s, only 27 per cent per cent of the UK population accessed regular dental care. The government were keen for this to improve, and launched health education campaigns, proclaiming in a 1944 report 'The British Public is ill educated and apathetic in regards to the care of the teeth. This attitude springs mainly from the national fear of pain and lack of any real understanding of the importance of dental health'. They were keen to change habits to encourage people to visit the dentist for regular inspections rather than when prompted by pain.

Water Fluoridisation

The use of fluoride proved one of the most effective public health improvements of the twentieth century in reducing tooth decay. Its discovery can be traced back to Colorado Springs, in 1908, when a local dentist noticed that people living in this area has less decay than those in the neighbouring villages. Analysis of the water supply showed high levels of fluoride. Artificial fluoridation of water supply was introduced in the states in 1945, and trialled in the UK, in Birmingham in 1964. Fluoride based toothpastes were launched in the early 1960's, and mass scale production followed in the 1970's.

Toothbrush Drill at School – England circa 1920. (From the Wellcome Collection)

NHS Dentistry

When dental care was included in NHS provisions in 1948, demand for treatment was overwhelming. Reports spoke of dentists seeing over a hundred patients a day as people flocked in to sort out their previously neglected not so pearly whites. Surgeries were open seven days a week, and patients still had to be turned away. At the end of the first year, many dentists were earning £4000 a year after expenses (compared to roughly £1400 before 1948 – and almost double that of the average family doctor during the same period). Restrictions were later introduced to reduce pay-outs over a specified level.

Prior to free dental treatment, it was common to be given a set of dentures as a wedding present – patients would have all of their teeth extracted in favour of a complete set of fake choppers, which avoided multiple future trips to the dentist. In the first nine months of the NHS, 33 million sets of artificial teeth had been provided by NHS dentists. Everyone wanted a pair. Not just one pair – often two, or three sets since they weren't paying for them. This figure had reached 66 million between 1950 and 1951, putting such a drain on the NHS, that the first charges were introduced.

Charges have increased since then, and various service re-organisations have taken place, resulting in an NHS service in which patients have to contribute towards the cost of care. Some dentists remarked that they had never been a part of the NHS in the same way as GPs, who received capitation payments for all patients registered on their lists, while dentists were contractors who were paid on a fee for service basis.

As of April 2019, there are three standard charges for all NHS dental treatments in England and Wales:

- Band 1 course of treatment – £22.70 in England, £14.70 in Wales; covers an examination, diagnosis (including X-rays), advice on how to prevent future problems, a scale and polish if needed, and application of fluoride varnish or fissure sealant. Band 1 also covers emergency care needed for trauma and severe pain or swelling, even if more than one visit is required.
- Band 2 course of treatment – £62.10 in England (Wales: £47.00) covers everything listed in Band 1, plus fillings, root canal work or removal of teeth.
- Band 3 course of treatment – £269.30 (Wales: £203.00) covers everything listed in Bands 1 and 2, plus crowns, dentures and bridges.

NHS Dental examinations are free in Scotland. Patients are required to meet 80 per cent of the costs of additional treatment to a maximum of £384, unless exempt (see https://www.scottishdental.org/public/treatment-charges/). Dentists are paid in 'Units of Dental Activity', typical values being £20-35. They are paid one UDA for a band 1 course of treatment, three for a band 2, and twelve for a band 3 course of treatment. Patient charges are deducted from these values meaning that for many treatments, the rate of pay is below the cost of actually providing the treatment and as a result, many dentists will refer patients elsewhere for treatments that will not provide them with a profit.

In 2016, the British Dental Association (BDA) released figures showing that dental charges had pushed 600,000 patients with dental problems to see already overstretched GPs, unequipped to provide dental treatment, costing £26 million in wasted GP appointments. One in five patients had reportedly postponed dental treatment due to concerns about costs and based on the current trajectory of dental charge increases, it is estimated that by the year 2032, patient charges will actually exceed the funding provided by the government in the NHS dental budget.

It is a sad fact that the NHS has betrayed its founding principles and is simply not free at the point of use for dental care, resulting in a service that is isolating many patients. Charities such as Dentaid now operate in some parts of the UK to provide free care where dental waiting lists are long and people are unable to access NHS dentists. The state of NHS finances means that the rest of healthcare is in danger of suffering the same fate.

My NHS Story

Kate Cavanagh is a UK Veterinary Surgeon and reflects on her experiences of customers paying for care for their pets

'Most veterinary care throughout the developed world is given through private practices owned by individuals or partners. Prices vary due to area, experience of staff, amenities and reputation but are largely in the control of the owner(s). In recent years corporate chains have surfaced, buying out many of the independent practices and bringing a more standardised pricing system. I qualified as a Veterinary Surgeon 15 years ago. For many years I worked as an assistant at various private practices in the UK around the Northwest and Midlands.

'You may wonder what this has to do with the NHS. Eight years ago, I moved to a niche area of our profession – the charity sector. I would like to share with you some of my personal reasons for this switch, and how I see similarities between the veterinary sector and medical sector. Perhaps lessons can be learnt from the smaller-scale veterinary profession.

'I work for a charity aiming to serve those on the bottom financial rung of UK society. We encourage donations for treatment, but it is effectively free treatment at the point of service, similar to the NHS. To our clients, our service is often seen as a sort of NHS for their pets. However, we are entirely charity financed, mainly through the giving of legacies and have no government funding. I guess you could say, like the NHS, we are spending other people's money, so are duty bound to make best use of it.

'Throughout my career in private practice I was exposed to what I can only describe as the monetisation of life and death. Pet insurance is not mandatory. Owners who do not have insurance (or have insurance that does not cover that situation or have it perhaps where the limit has been reached), are faced with the daunting prospect that they may not be able to afford treatment for their pet. Consultations can be a relentless battle between what we should do and what we can do. Discussions regarding costs can take the limelight instead of the animal. The challenge of trying to maintain clinical standards and integrity whilst staying within each owner's budget was often the hardest aspect of the job. It could end in following a treatment route that is far from ideal, or ultimately, premature euthanasia of the pet on financial grounds.

'A case I remember well was that of a young Yorkshire Terrier named Betty. She was forever trying to make friends with the neighbour's cat. The feeling was not mutual, and after the most recent altercation, a scratch on her eye developed into an ulcer. It did not respond well to treatment and in the end the only option was to remove the eye. Even at a very heavily discounted price (zero profit) the owner could still not finance it, and at a later date she was euthanised. An awful situation for that pet owner and the vet involved, knowing that something could be done but finances prevented it. Not charging appropriately may ease the conscience but the business would not last long.

'Situations like that of Betty can cause feelings of guilt and anger. I have heard colleagues being called murderers and face verbal and physical abuse. Occasionally we personally take on the animals and associated costs using our own money. Many vets end up with a 'rescue', which are often three-legged, or one-eyed, or missing something! Sadly, this cannot be the case every time. The toll on vets, who are often deeply compassionate and caring people, and the ones holding that last needle, is often forgotten.

'The daily struggle with situations like this was part of why I left private practice to work in the charity sector. As a doey eyed, animal loving, James Herriot addicted, 12 year old, I had not thought about this side of the job. Of course, in my current job we have to make sensible decisions with our funds, I suppose in the same way the NHS does. But clinical standards are good and Betty's situation would never happen. We treat dozens of animals just like her every day. I wonder in the USA and other countries, where there is a limited social medical care system, how many difficult decisions patients, relatives and doctors have to make due to finances. Thanks to the NHS it is an added angle that we don't have to worry about. The prospect of that changing scares me. It is traumatic having these discussions over a much loved pet but imagine if a similar scenario played out at your next appointment in the GP or with a doctor about a sick relative. Unimaginable.

'The subject of veterinary bills comes up a lot, many telling me how astounded they are at bills they receive for veterinary care. I wonder if many consider the cost of their own healthcare. If so, would they find vets' bills so shocking? Prices do vary nationally, but at my local private veterinary practice a consultation with medication costs around £50-60. I don't know what the equivalent GP consult with medicine costs. Perhaps we should all know the answer to this.* Vets often use similar equipment and medicines, often sending samples to the same laboratories for testing. I remember, during my university days before MRI scanners were commonplace in veterinary medicine, lurking behind the human MRI scanner on Crown Street in Liverpool waiting for the humans to leave before we could use the scanner for our furry patients. Do people know how much an MRI scan costs? An X-ray? A course of physiotherapy? I hear complaints about prescription charges. If the real cost of the medicine people are taking were known, perhaps they would consider it a steal. Expectations and longevity have increased, with more people wanting 'Supervet' style treatment without the price tag. Perhaps this is true of my counterparts in the medical profession.

'We price up the work we perform, as we would for a paying client, and present this itemised 'dummy' bill to the client. It gives them an

---

* According to the Personal Social Services Research Unit (PSSRU) the cost of an 11.7 minute face to face GP consultation (excluding direct care staff costs and without qualification costs) in 2015 was £33. http://www.pssru.ac.uk/project-pages/unit-costs/2017

idea of how much the care of their pet would have cost, were they not eligible to use our service. The aim being to raise awareness of veterinary costs and also encourage donations. Perhaps doing this for healthcare would help raise awareness of how much our healthcare really costs. It would also help people see that veterinary charges are fair.

'I feel hugely grateful to have a National Health Service, and to those that work to keep it grinding on day by day. Perhaps I have seen in some small way some of the effects privatisation would have for patients and workers. I will continue to both celebrate it and protect it with pride wherever I can. Although we already have many fabulous human medical charities to cover gaps in funding, I suppose without a National Health Service style system, charities like my own would be needed to rescue those on that bottom financial rung of society.'

A Different World: 1948 vs 2018

When the NHS began in 1948, the UK population stood at 49.4 million. 70 years later in 2018, the population is estimated at 66.5 million. By 2068 this is predicted to grow to 82 million. There are an estimated 3million people with diabetes in England, and 26 per cent per cent of both men and women are now classified as obese. The population is expected to continue to age with the number of people over 60 expected to rise from 14.9m in 2014 to 21.9m by 2039 – all which will have implications for healthcare.

- Life expectancy – In 1948 the life expectancy for men was 66 and for women, 71. Today, men can expect to live to the age of 79.2 and women 82.9
- Infant mortality – In 1948 there were 34.5 deaths per 1000 live births. Today that figure is 3.7
- Death – In 1948, the main killers were rheumatic heart disease (almost unheard of today) circulatory disorders and infection. Over the past 70 years, the proportion of deaths caused by cancer has risen (in line with an aging population), while those caused by tuberculosis and respiratory disease have fallen.

- In 1948, 65 per cent per cent of Britain's population smoked. Figures from 2013 show that this number has dropped to less than 20 per cent per cent
- In 1948, the annual cost of the NHS per head, per lifetime was £200. Today that figure has risen to £2106
- The NHS was launched with 68,013 hospital staff (excluding doctors). In March 2017, the NHS employed 106,430 doctors, 285,893 nurses, 21,597 midwives, 132,673 technical staff, 19,772 ambulance staff, 21,139 managers and 9974 senior managers
- In 1950, there were approximately 21,450 GPs in Britain. In March 2017 there were 33,423 full time GPs (excluding locums) – a reduction of 890 from 2016
- Today, the NHS sees 1 million patients every 36 hours

Chapter 3

Timeline of the NHS

1950s

The first decade of the NHS was not without its problems, but it was successful enough to cement it into an institution. A free, universal service was a huge cultural change from what had preceded it, and only three years into the NHS, financial challenges became evident resulting in the introduction of charges for prescriptions, dental and optical services by the end of 1952. The fifties saw a post war baby boom and the introduction of technologies such as the microwave oven, plastics, nylon stockings and computers. Medical technological also thrived. Ultrasound was adapted for use in foetal monitoring and the success of antibiotics in the 1940s was followed by a rash of new drugs. Cortisone was discovered in 1950 as were the thiazides for hypertension and the first effective remedies for tuberculosis were introduced. Antipsychotics such as chlorpromazine and haloperidol were synthesised, the use of blood products became more common and interferon was discovered. The Thalidomide tragedy started in 1958, when pregnant women were prescribed the medication as a tranquilliser – only to find in the 1960s that it was responsible for causing severe birth defects. In 1954, in the USA, the food preservative BHA (butylated hydroxyanisole) was approved (the same year that McDonalds was franchised) signalling the growth of fast food chains, ready-made meals and the start of the obesity epidemic.

1950   **The link between smoking and lung cancer is proven.** Richard
        Doll had been studying lung cancer patients since the 1940s,
        expecting to find it was caused by fumes from coal fires or
        cars, but instead found that smokers are more likely to die
        of lung cancer than non-smokers. He also found an increased
        risk of heart disease. Doll quit smoking during his study and
        lived to the age of 92.

The Dangers of Smoking. (Taken from the Wellcome Collection)

The Collings Report – the first major report on quality in general practice – found poor standards of care, poor working conditions and isolation from other professionals. GPs had remained outside of the NHS as independent contractors rather than salaried employees. The 1948 NHS Act had intended that GPs would move away from being single handed, and would be rehoused with other GPs inside health centres, but this proved unaffordable.
Labour Government

1951   **Charges for dental and optical appliances imposed**
          Conservative Government

1952   **Prescription charges** of one shilling are introduced and a flat rate of £1 for ordinary dental treatment
          College of General Practitioners formed
          Watson and Crick discover structure of DNA (Deoxyribonucleic acid). DNA makes up our genes, which pass on hereditary characteristics from parent to child. Knowing their structure set the foundations for the study of genetic diseases.

DNA double helix. (Peter Artymiuk, Wellcome Collection)

1953 Coronation of Queen Elizabeth II

Summit of Everest climbed for the first time by Sir Edmund Hillary and Tenzing Norgay

1954 Children are granted daily visits from their families while in hospital. Until this time, visiting was only permitted for an hour at the weekend. Children were often placed alone in adult wards, with little explanation as to what was happening to them. Paediatricians realised that this separation was traumatic and instituted family visiting.

Rationing ends

The Percy Commission is established by Winston Churchill's government to review the care given to people with mental health problems. They recommend that treatment should be given in the community where possible, rather than in large

NHS Prescription Stamps (via Wikimedia Commons)

psychiatric institutions. This is supported by the 1959 Mental Health Act, which also states that mentally ill patients should not be differentiated from physically sick patients.

1956 **The Guillebaud Report** on the cost of the NHS is published. It reports that the cost of the NHS in relative terms is falling and that capital spending is 33 per cent per cent of pre-war levels and that future costs would be met by economic growth.

The Clean Air Act is passed, aimed at reducing the air pollution created by burning coal. In 1952, a 'Great Smog' descended upon London, exacerbating the health problems of those with heart and lung conditions, resulting in a dramatic increase in mortality rates. The act allowed local authorities to control emissions from industrial premises and improved death rates.

1957 **The Willick Report** suggests a 12 per cent per cent reduction in the number of doctors being trained, due to the increasing numbers of specialist registrars unable to secure specialist

(© Telegraph Media Group Limited)

consultant posts. This is later considered a misjudgement, and training numbers are increased in 1961. The report is retrospectively believed to be responsibility for the severe shortages of junior medical staff throughout the 1960s.

1958   **Polio and Diptheria vaccination programme launched** ensuring everyone under 15 years is vaccinated, leading to a dramatic reduction in cases
        The Opticians Act allows opticians to become regulated professionals

My NHS Story

Meg Parkes is an Honorary Research Fellow at the Liverpool School of Tropical Medicine. She trained as a nurse in the 1970s and reflects on her NHS experiences

'I was born into the NHS in 1953: I was 0, it was nearly 5. I grew up in it, the daughter of two General Practitioners who worked tirelessly for the benefit of others. It helped to shape me. After leaving school, I first trained as a medical secretary and then applied to train as a general nurse. During the secretarial course I gained a broader understanding of the local NHS services – GPs' surgeries, local clinics and administration.

'I began three years of adult State Registered Nurse (SRN) training in September 1972 at Manchester Royal Infirmary (MRI). It was an apprenticeship and we had to live-in for the first year of training; all uniform was provided – cotton dresses, cuffs, collars, caps and capes and of course, starched aprons – and laundered by the hospital. Nurses' Homes were run by wardens and we had single rooms off long, deep carpeted corridors (to ensure quiet for those on night duty) at the end of which were the bathrooms, each with cast iron baths the size of small troop carriers. The hot water was never ending... what bliss!

'Pre-NHS the MRI had been a voluntary hospital (funded by public subscription), the city's premier university teaching hospital. An air of excellence pervaded the wards and its endless miles of corridors; those of us accepted for training were encouraged to feel part of an elite and were expected to maintain the reputation and dignity of the hospital. I certainly felt very privileged to be there. After an eight-week introductory course we nurse chicks were let loose on unsuspecting wards full of patients. This was where our apprenticeships really began, learning from the senior student nurses and qualified staff by observing, before eventually being allowed to try. In between times we took temperatures and cleaned anything that stood still. Our 12-week placements included time in medicine, surgery, orthopaedics and gynaecology – each followed by two-week blocks, known as School, where we had lectures and practical training.

'My first month's salary, with tax, NI and living-in charges deducted, was £48. For this I had worked five eight-hour day shifts per week. Early shifts started at 7.30am, lates at 12.30pm, with the dreaded split shifts – in at 7.30am, off at 1pm, back in at 4pm till 9pm – whenever the rota dictated. After just six months' training we were eligible for the night rota: 11-hour shifts from 9pm – 8am worked over a fortnight. It was common to work 10 nights on followed by four off. Though responsibility on nights was enormous we survived, as did most of our patients.

'On qualifying and promotion to staff nurse, we were expected to work at the hospital for at least a further year to earn our Hospital Badge (at MRI this was a large, distinctive and much-coveted bronze penny). Regrettably it was not for me. Due to ill-health, I had to defer my training for 18 months and spent time working as the manager of a General Practice, seeing the NHS from a different perspective.

'I eventually completed my training at what were then known as Hope Hospital and Salford Royal, and came to realise this change of hospitals helped broaden my outlook. Hope Hospital was, pre-NHS, a municipal hospital (former Poor Law, or Work House hospital). It was more 'local' than MRI in every sense – patients, staff, nursing experience. While serious or unusual cases were routinely referred to MRI, there was still plenty of acute medicine and surgery to keep us busy.

'One stark memory of my student days was that we were always rushed off our feet. We never felt we had enough time to give our patients the care we knew they needed. Wards were often short staffed, especially during winters and compromise was the order of the day: 'prioritise the urgent and do the best you can for the rest' was a constant mantra. We felt really embattled at times. Sound familiar?

'Another lasting memory was when, towards the end of my first year, I got engaged. I was summoned before MRI's formidable Matron, a highly-acclaimed nurse with a fearsome reputation. She quizzed me about my determination to complete my training, told me that the hospital's needs were my priority and whether I got the day off to get married was entirely in the hands of the sister in charge of the ward! I did, but only because I had temporarily left training. I knew one student who worked a split shift on her wedding day.

'After qualifying I worked briefly, as a staff nurse on nights at a local general hospital. I vividly remember on one shift, a boorish patient berating me for being late to answer a patient's bell. Myself and an auxiliary (healthcare assistant) were busy at the other end of the ward and I had responded as soon as I could. The man loudly demanded better service for himself and his fellow patients, ending his rant by stating dramatically, "I pay my stamp. I am entitled to a proper service, it's my right!" I looked him in the eye and said calmly, "Your stamp won't buy the floor tile you're standing on." As I walked across to the patient who had really needed my attention applause broke out around me.

'I look back on my all too brief years of nursing with gratitude for such a valuable training for life. What a privilege it is to care for others when they are most in need. Having four children put paid to my return to nursing, shifts even in the late 1980s were not family friendly.

'Now in my mid-60s, I believe my generation has been the most fortunate in every sense: born into a country that was free, with free education, healthcare, almost unlimited choices and the chance of a decent pension. We should remember that. Stop moaning about 'the broken NHS', give thanks and do something useful, like paying for services when we can afford to, so it can work better. What finer legacy could we leave our families.'

1960s

The buoyant economy of the technicolour sixties brought low unemployment rates and increasing affluence. UK families bought their first cars, kitchen appliances and televisions, and mass communication became a reality. Music and fashion defined the era, and rebellious lyrics against the authorities fostered young people to stand up for their beliefs and individuality. Sixties teenagers were the first generation free from conscription and the decade saw laws regarding divorce, homosexuality and abortion become more liberalised. Feminism gained credibility meaning women could broaden their dreams beyond motherhood and marriage. In 1968, 850 female factory workers in Dagenham went on strike, fighting for equal pay to their male co-workers – and the Equal Pay Act was passed in 1970 as a result. The newly introduced contraceptive pill created a sexual revolution, while a boom in pharmaceuticals saw the development of drugs of abuse: Valium to soothe the nerves of housewives, and psychotropic drugs such as LSD which helped bring about the 'hippie' movement. Immigration brought with it foreign imports such as spaghetti Bolognese and chicken tikka masala, forever changing the nation's eating habits. Immigration also bolstered the workforce of the NHS. The Caribbean and Ireland had been a primary source of nurses since the 1940s, in the 1960s more than 18,000 doctors came from Indian and Pakistan in response to an appeal by health minister Enoch Powell. NHS inefficiencies were apparent in the sixties and a system of health authorities was proposed to replace the disjointed tripartite system; this eventually came into being in the seventies.

1960 **Male nurses** are admitted to the Royal College of Nursing for the first time. When registration for nurses was introduced in 1919, trained male nurses (who often worked in asylums) were not able to join and were kept on a supplementary register until 1960.

Surgical Firsts. The first successful UK living kidney transplant is performed by Michael Woodruff in Edinburgh. The 49-year-old twins both survive for six years, before dying of an unrelated illness. In the same year, the first full hip replacement is carried out at the Wrightington Hospital by Professor John Charnley.

Pelvic xray showing a total hip joint replacement, (via Wikimedia Commons)

He asks patients if they mind returning their hips to him post mortem; and the majority agree, allowing him to check for wear and tear and research improved future models.

1961   **The oral contraceptive pill is launched**, and is hailed as a twentieth century breakthrough, playing a role in liberating women and enabling greater sexual freedom. For the first time, sex was effectively separated from reproduction; allowing childbirth to be planned around careers, resulting in a reduction in early marriages, and increase in female university enrolment. It has prompted both health scares and moral debates since its introduction. Initially it is only offered to married women, but this is relaxed in 1967, and by 1969, almost 1 million women are using it. Provision of contraception was initially the work of charitable organisations such as the Family Planning Association and Marie Stopes, but once it became available on NHS prescription, patients increasingly obtained it from their GP. All forms of contraception remain free in the UK today on the NHS. Patients in the USA can pay up to $50 per month for birth control pills and up to $1300 to have an intrauterine contraceptive device (IUD) inserted.

Enoch Powell's Water Tower Speech is seen as a milestone in mental health service provision, speaking of an end to the old asylums and a move to greater community care

The oral contraceptive pill. (Beria L Rodriguez via Wikipedia Commons)

1962   The Hospital Plan approved the development of District General Hospitals for populations of around 125,000; in an attempt to unify the tripartite system of hospitals, GPs and local authorities, and make hospitals accessible to the populations they served. A ten year construction plan is put in place. New hospitals had not been built for many years prior to this and the costs and time involved in the redevelopment were grossly underestimated at the outset.

The Porritt Review is published the same year, led by old-school surgeon Sir Arthur Porritt. He was initially sceptical about the formation of NHS (and had been a critic in the 1940s), but had been convinced that it had to continue. He suggested the system was fragmented, and that Area Health Boards should be established to bring together hospital, GP and community services.

1964   Water Fluoridation is introduced to the water supply with the intention to reduce tooth decay
Labour government

1965   Prescription charges abolished
Abolition of the Death Penalty
The Seebohm Committee is established and later publish their report in 1968 reviewing the organisation and responsibilities of the social services functions of the local authorities. They advise an amalgamation of welfare services, home help, mental health and social work services to create a unified department, able to support care in the community.

1966   A new contract improved pay and conditions for GPs, instituting a maximum list size of 2,000 patients, improving resources available for professional education and improvement in premises and hiring support staff. Following this, group practices became the norm.

1967   The Salmon Report makes recommendations for developing the nursing staff structure and the status of the profession in hospital management.
The Cogwheel Report considers the organization of doctors within hospitals and proposes speciality groupings
The Abortion Act is introduced by the Liberal MP David Steel and becomes law in 1968, allowing termination of pregnancy by a registered physician up to 28 weeks gestation, if two other

doctors agree that it is in the best mental and physical interests of the woman. In 1990, this is reduced to 24 weeks. Abortion was only decriminalised in Northern Ireland in October 2019, with a framework for lawful abortion services coming into effect in March 2020.

1968   **Britain's first heart transplant** is carried out in May 1968 by South African born surgeon Donald Ross in London. A team of eighteen spend seven hours on the procedure; on what is the tenth procedure of its kind carried out since the operation was pioneered by Christiaan Barnard in Cape Town, a year earlier. The patient dies after 46 days from an associated infection
Sextuplets born. After undergoing fertility treatment, a British woman gives birth to four girls and two boys at Birmingham maternity hospital, assisted by a team of twenty-eight. One of the girls dies at the birth and two more die later.
Prescription charges reintroduced
The first green paper on the NHS is published, recommending the creation of 50 area boards in attempt to remedy the organisational deficiencies of the NHS. Governmental Green papers are typically consultation papers containing proposals for change, while White Papers are issued as statements of policy and often set out changes for new legislation – known as

Pro-abortion protestors. (©Marx
Memorial Library/Mary Evans)

Group of surgeons in the operating room. (Adobe Stock Images)

a Bill, which is then debated in Parliament. When a Bill is given Royal Assent by the Queen, it becomes an Act – and thus Law. It is often enacted a year after it passes through Parliament.

The Department of Health and Social Security is formed from the merging of the Ministry of Health and the Ministry of Social Security

1969   **Man on the moon** – Buzz Aldrin and Neil Armstrong become the first men to step on the moon

The Liverpool School of Tropical Medicine and Far East Prisoners of War

The Liverpool School of Tropical Medicine (LSTM) had a long post-war collaboration with British ex-Far East Prisoners of War (FEPOWs). These men suffered from the consequences of captivity for decades after their release, many of them still experiencing relapses of amoebic dysentery and malaria many years later. From 1968 until 1999, LSTM was asked by the Department of Health to become the primary centre

Liverpool School of Tropical Medicine in 1951 — Wikimedia commons for these veterans to undergo Tropical Disease Investigations (TDIs). Far East veterans were often referred by their GPs, or sometimes even self-referred, but the majority of men were sent to Liverpool by the Ministry of Pensions as a result of an application for a war pension. The DHSS funded travel costs and pensions when they were awarded, with the programme becoming big enough to establish a FEPOW Unit at the DHSS offices in the 1980s. The Tropical School was not an NHS institution, but these men were assessed in NHS beds run by the school and attended to by physicians who were university employed and had honorary NHS Consultant Physician contracts. Many doctors were involved, but the vast majority of TDIs were undertaken by Dr Dion Bell, who saw hundreds of FEPOWs which led to him achieving an iconic status among the FEPOW community. In the 1970s, Dr Geoff Gill (now Emeritus Professor of International Medicine) became involved, mainly in the research side until the last TDI took place in 1999. As well as providing clinical care, LSTM doctors and scientists made advances in laboratory diagnostic tests for conditions such as *Strongyloides stercoralis* (a parasitic infection caused by a nematode worm). They conducted detailed studies into the long-term health effects of Far East captivity and the problems suffered by this group such as chronic neuropathic syndromes, mental health problems (now recognised as PTSD) and persistent strongyloidiasis.

In more recent years, the LSTM Far East POW project moved to medical historical enquiries into the POW experience, including a major oral history project led by Meg Parkes, in which 67 veterans and 10 wives and widows shared their stories of captivity, survival and the post-war aftermath. Extracts of these interviews and more about Liverpool's FEPOW project can be found here: www.captivememories.org.uk.

My NHS Story

Professor Geoff Gill, Consultant Physician at Aintree University Hospital, and Emeritus Professor of International Medicine at the University of Liverpool reflects on his time in the NHS between 1973 and 2018:

'I qualified in medicine at the University of Newcastle-upon-Tyne and began work for the NHS as a house physician in 1973. Apart from just over three years working abroad, I worked in the NHS continually until finally "hanging up my stethoscope" in early 2018 – a total of 42 years. This included 20 years (1996-2016) as a clinical academic (half university and half NHS), and a few years post-retirement part-time work.

'My leaning was always towards hospital rather than primary care work, and I trained in medicine, becoming a consultant physician (specialising in diabetes and endocrinology) in 1985. The training jobs in those days were house doctor, senior house officer (SHO), registrar, senior registrar and finally consultant. Rotational jobs were only just coming in when I started, and doctors (particularly at SHO level) often took one-off six or 12 month positions. This gave less job security than nowadays but did give some degree of training flexibility. You very much "learnt on the job", and there was nothing like today's system of educational supervisors or on-line training records. However, I do remember that as a senior registrar I met with a regional committee once a year to check on progress and breadth of experience etc. – pretty informal but in some ways more effective than current on-line "box-ticking"!

'The loss of the senior registrar (SR) grade was I think a great shame. This was technically four years but often much longer, and in the medical specialities almost every SR took two years out to do research and write up an MD thesis. Towards the end of the SR grade, you very much acted as a junior consultant. I recall doing a six-month locum consultant physician job in Gateshead in my final SR year. Newly appointed consultant physicians in those days were much more able to cope with their new duties and responsibilities.

'Working hours have thankfully reduced from the crazy on-call systems of the 1970s and before. Working weeks of over 100 hours were not uncommon, frequently working a whole day, then on-call for a night, and working the following day also. To be fair, there was much less to do in the way of treatment and investigation, and the number of emergency admissions was significantly smaller than today. We also often covered our own ward only, without emergency "take" duties. Overall, we operated very much as a "firm" with full continuity of care from admission to discharge. Good though this was, I can't see it possible to go back to such a system with the present volume of admissions and limits on junior doctor working hours.

'When I began work in the 1970s, the ward medical system was almost feudal. Consultants were god-like people, with a strict pecking order down the grades below them. Consultant ward rounds were incredibly important affairs, attended by the whole medical firm, and almost always the ward sister. The patient was not expected to make comments or ask questions! In fact, the general lack of patient involvement in those days was quite incredible. Part of this was the culture of the times, and the public were very respectful and deferential to the medical profession. If a diagnosis of cancer was made, patients were often not told, and words like "inflammation" were used. I remember being quite uncomfortable with this practice, though I suspect the patients concerned eventually guessed what was the matter with them.

'The loss of nursing input from our medical ward rounds in recent years has been very regrettable, but overall modern team-based and patient-centred care has been welcome. My later work was mostly on our hospital's Acute Medical Unit, and we were constantly inter-acting with a multitude of healthcare professionals – nurses, pharmacists, physiotherapists, occupational therapists, speech therapists – all on an equal professional basis.

'Politics has to be mentioned, of course, and my career has sadly seen increasing political interference with the running of the NHS from central government. "Reforms" and "consultations" cost a lot of money and rarely improve care. Wheels are constantly being re-invented, and levels of command altered but basic underlying problems remain unanswered – for example overall underfunding, separation of health and social care, and lack of adequately planned workforce numbers.

'Despite all this, some things have not changed. Faced with a sick patient, I have always had the same interaction and communication, using the time honoured skills of history, examination and investigation. And when the assessment was complete, I could do what we physicians should always do: "cure sometimes, help often, support always".'

1970s

The seventies was a decade of strikes – miners, dustmen, postal workers – and financial problems. For most ordinary people, the seventies brought experiences that their grandparents could never have imagined – cheap air travel meant package holidays abroad became common and 91 per cent per cent of people had a (often colour) television. The NHS saw real advances in medical progress. CT scans and transplants became available and the first computers found their way into NHS hospitals. The organisation of the NHS continued to be debated and a new system of Area and Regional health authorities was implemented in 1974 to try to distribute resources more evenly. This was criticised for being too complicated and too top heavy with managers. In the mid-1970s, then health secretary Barbara Castle tried to phase out private patients being treated in NHS facilities. The decade ended with Britain's first female Prime Minister Margaret Thatcher coming into power, and worldwide eradication of smallpox was achieved through vaccination.

1970   **NHS Reorganisation.** The second Green Paper on the NHS rejects the idea of local authorities managing the health service and the debate opens again about the reorganising of the NHS **Conservative government**

1972   **CT Scans introduced.** Computer tomography scans were invented in the late 1960s by Sir Godfrey Hounsfield and became commercially viable in 1972. They revolutionised medical imaging, allowing doctors to see three dimensional views inside the body without performing surgery.
       The Cochrane Report sets out the vital importance of randomised controlled trials in assessing the effectiveness of treatments, leading the way for evidence-based medicine
       The Royal College of General Practitioners is established giving GPs an official representative body for the first time.

1973   **The NHS Reorganisation Act** (preceded by a 1972 White Paper) sees the traditional tripartite structure replaced in an attempt to generate better co-ordination between health authorities and local authorities. Under the reforms, regional

CT Scanner
(Weezie23
via Wikimedia
Commons)

hospital boards are replaced by regional, area and district health authorities, which take over public health and other services (vaccination, health visiting, epidemiological work) from the local authorities. Family planning becomes part of the NHS for the first time. Environmental health and some health education remains a local government responsibility, while the duties of the medical officers for health are transferred to the NHS.

1974   **Labour Government**
The Role of Medical Officer of Health (the official charged with public health responsibilities) is abolished and the duties divided between community physicians and local government health services. The decline in infectious disease (due to vaccinations and antibiotics) led to government reorganisations – but this was the start of the fragmentation of public health.

1975   **The Merrison Report** extends the functions of the GMC (in relation to medical education) to make them more accountable. Disciplinary processes are separated so those whose performances are impaired by ill health are recognised. It is suggested that doctors might undertake some sort of periodic 'relicensure', but the committee decided this was beyond its remit (Revalidation is eventually implemented in 2012 after a series of high profile medical scandals).
Endorphins are discovered by John Hughes and Hans Kosterlitz at the University of Aberdeen. These polypeptide substances are produced in the brain and resemble opiates in their ability to relieve pain thus working as natural painkillers.

1976   **The Resource Allocation Working Party** attempts to address the inequalities between health spending in the South East of England, and the lower levels spent elsewhere. It examines mortality in each area as an indicator of health need and manages from 1977-90 to redistribute resources to the poorer northern regions. 'Cash Limits' are introduced whereby spending authorities cannot exceed the sums of money allocated to them.
Mandatory training of GPs. Three-year postgraduate training programmes for GPs become mandatory

1978   **The world's first IVF baby is born.** Gynaecologist Patrick Steptoe and physiologist Robert Edward develop a technique to fertilise an egg outside the women's body before placing it in the womb, known as in vitro fertilisation. Louise Brown is the first 'test tube baby' to be born using this technique. Since then, more than a million children have been born this way worldwide

The Winter of Discontent caused by the oil crisis sees a worsening of the NHS's financial problems

The declaration of Alma Ata calls for urgent action by all governments to protect and promote health. It emphasises the role of primary care in carrying out public health duties such as immunisation, controlling and preventing epidemics, family planning and promoting health and nutrition.

1979   **First bone marrow transplant** is performed on a child with primary immunodeficiency at Great Ormond Street Hospital by Professor Roland Levinsky. Bone marrow helps create the body's immune system and today, the Antony Nolan Trust recruits bone marrow donors for those who suffer with diseases such as leukaemia and non-Hodgkins lymphoma.

Wearing seat belts made compulsory for drivers and front seat passengers in a car.

Conservative Government

Council house tennants given the right to buy their own home.

My NHS Story

Sister Judith Susser started her State Registered Nurse training at the Manchester Royal Infirmary (MRI) in 1972 and continued working in the NHS until recently. She shares her thoughts on her 45 year career:

'In retrospect I was very naive when I started my training and not politically minded so I therefore took the NHS for granted and never gave the organisation a second thought – I just wanted to survive from placement to placement and qualify.

'In brief, I qualified and worked as a staff nurse at MRI for 6 months, then went to Israel for 1 year as a volunteer nurse working in Beer Sheva in their (rudimentary) ITU. On return to the UK I worked privately in The Convent Nursing Home in Nottingham before going to do a Urology and Nephrology course at The 3 P's [Footnote - The three P's is the name given to the hospital group comprised of St Phillip's, St Peter's and St Paul's – which closed in 1992] in London. I worked there from 1977, moving to the Middlesex Hospital, then UCLH.

'For the last 15 years I have worked on the Spinal Cord Injury Centre at the Royal National Orthopaedic Hospital in Stanmore. In this specialised rehabilitation setting I am proud to say that there is total holistic care involving rehabilitation physicians, surgeons, neuro-physiologists, physiotherapists, OTs, dieticians, psychologists, psychiatrists, tissue viability teams, speech and language specialists, community liaison workers, fertility specialists, urologists and bowel care teams. The patients are with us from 3 months to 1 year and remain under our care for the rest of their lives. THIS is the NHS at its finest.

'I was so young and simple when I started at MRI. I had never seen anyone naked, or drunk, or indeed both at the same time! I was totally impressionable, and in awe of anyone senior to me, which was everyone. Terrifyingly I don't recall being phased by my total lack of knowledge, and I never questioned or queried anything. Questioning was not then in my nature, and I suspect it was not encouraged. Donning the complicated uniform gave me the confidence to face the world, but I was probably a total liability.

'After an introductory 6-8 weeks we were let loose on the wards. There was a lot of bed-making, bed baths, bedpan and urinal "rounds".

When patients returned from the operating theatre, after an hour or so they had a "post-op" wash. This comprised washing hands and face with a flannel, checking the dressings, swapping theatre gown for a nightie, changing the draw sheet and giving a mouth wash. The draw sheet was about one yard wide and was placed over a rubber sheet, (later to be superseded by plastic) under the patient's bottom. This was to save the necessity of changing the bottom bed sheet, probably not ideal for tissue viability.... all those potential creases and wrinkles. I believe the post-op wash does not exist anymore as so many procedures are now day cases. Nevertheless, it "freshened up" the patient, allowed assessment of their pain and general condition, and was an excellent example of old fashioned bedside care, that was most likely very welcome.

'Tasks were allocated as "rounds" to be completed. The "back" round involved taking a trolley from bed to bed giving pressure area care. Some patients were in bed for many days, but I do not remember seeing any pressure sores, so this must have been effective. My favourite round, being of an organised disposition, was "Obs". Again, with a trolley I went from bed to bed taking patient observations and completing their charts. Similarly, and just as enjoyable was doing the fluid In and Out charts. My charts were impeccable, but I'm ashamed to say I had no critical evaluation faculties, therefore a patient may have been haemorrhaging internally or seriously dehydrated and no alarm bells rang in my task driven skull.

'The first Christmas I experienced was lovely. The hospital was made up of long, narrow Nightingale wards. We were asked to sit with elderly patients, at their bedside. A choir of nurses led by the sisters, with their navy, red-lined capes worn inside-out, and carrying lanterns sang walking from ward to ward, the lights being dimmed. I remember with moving anticipation hearing the choir move from ward to ward.

'There was unfortunately some, what would now constitute institutional bullying. Looking back, the first bed-bath I was asked to perform alone was on an elderly male patient. I was told to wash, dress him and get him up. When I went behind the screens there was a prosthetic leg leaning up against the wall. My face must have been a picture! Then there was being sent to the stores department for both a "long stand" and a "dead weight". It surprises me that I'm not still stupidly standing there!

'We were in charge on night duty probably after 1 year in training. We worked with one or two nursing auxiliaries and were supervised by the night sister who covered many wards. I do not recall being aghast at this huge responsibility, as I would be now. Ah, the callowness of youth. I do remember the satisfaction of doing the late night drink round, Ovaltine or Horlicks, maybe a Mackeson, closing the blinds and dimming the lights and settling the patients down to sleep.

'One morning, as a staff nurse, I was giving out breakfast on my ward, which had been divided into 6 bed bays. I trundled my trolley round calling to the patients "porridge or flakes, hot milk or cold, sugar, tea or coffee?" One patient lay sleeping. I yelled these choices a couple of times, the other patients watching me. Eventually it dawned on me that he was not going to need breakfast that day, or ever again. I pulled the curtains round the bed and tried to compose my face prior to walking out past five pairs of knowing eyes.

'Nowadays, watching programmes such as 24 Hours in A&E, I say: "Thank God for the NHS." It seems to me that the more over-managed and beleaguered it becomes, the more these programmes proliferate. In my area of North Central London an external focus group gathered views and trends within the nursing workforce. They found a lack of new and younger staff climbing the ranks, and that among the nurses over 50 years of age, the majority were sticking around for financial reasons, rather than the joy of the job.

'I handed in my notice to retire, after another demeaning interaction with a manager, who wanted us to move office again in a reorganisation that made no sense, then said to me in a meeting, when I queried this, "I'm not asking you, I'm telling you." I still do my old job for two days a week on the "bank" (an internal hospital agency), until they advertise and fill my position, predictably at a lower grade.'

1980s

The eighties are remembered for big hair and shoulder pads, and the emergence of a frightening new disease – AIDS – which caused previously healthy people to die from rare conditions. The AIDS epidemic began in 1981, when unusual clusters of Pneumocystis carinii pneumonia were reported in homosexual men in Los Angeles. Homophobia was rife, and the disease was initially labelled GRID (Gay Related Immune Deficiency) until it was evident that half of those affected were not homosexual. The disease was poorly understood, and millions died until HIV was discovered as the cause and developments in immunology meant treatments started to become available. The eighties saw a rise in drug resistance – widespread use of antibiotics since the 1940s had allowed infectious organisms to adapt to become resistant, meaning the drugs used to kill them were no longer effective. There was a focus on preventative medicine in the eighties and a notion that individuals were responsible for their own health and lifestyle choices and breast and cervical screening programs were introduced to the NHS. Privatisation also took off in the eighties – with British Telecom, British Gas, British Steel and the Water Authorities (among others) all being affected. British Rail followed in the nineties. The NHS looked like it would follow suit when Margaret Thatcher announced plans to reform the NHS and introduce an internal market.

1980   **MRI (Magnetic Resonance Imaging) Scans** are introduced providing detailed information about the soft tissues of the body by using a combination of magnetism and radio frequency waves.
        Laparoscopic (Keyhole) Surgery is used for the first time to remove a gallbladder.

Laparoscopy operation (Abode Stock Images)

The Black Report, commissioned by the Labour Government in 1977, investigates inequalities in health, finding that those in lower socioeconomic groups suffer higher rates of mortality. Access to health services, particularly preventative services is poor among the working class. It recommends increased spending on community health and primary care, and government intervention with increased child benefits, improved housing and agreeing minimum working conditions with unions. The new conservative government did not endorse these recommendations due to the scale of expenditure involved.

1981 **First UK death from AIDS.** A 41-year-old man dies from an acquired immunodeficiency syndrome (AIDS) related illness in London. Terry Higgins was one of the first people to die of the disease a year later, leading to the formation of the Terrance Higgins Trust. By 1984, scientists had identified that human immunodeficiency virus (HIV) caused AIDS and testing was introduced in 1985. The 'Don't die of ignorance' public health campaign was launched in 1987. Triple combination therapy

World AIDS Day 1994 (Wellcome Collection)

(Highly active anti-retroviral therapy or HAART) became standard in 1996 and HIV treatment became free for everyone in England in 2012. The term AIDS describes a set of illnesses people with HIV can get if they don't receive treatment. In the 1980s, HIV treatment wasn't so good and most people would eventually succumb to these diseases. Today, treatment is so good that few people develop AIDS. People newly diagnosed with HIV today can expect a normal life expectancy, if they have timely diagnosis and treatment. The landmark PARTNER study recently showed that people with HIV who are on effective treatment to suppress their viral load, cannot pass HIV on to others. In August 2017, NHS England started a trial of HIV prevention drugs (Pre-exposure prophylaxis or PrEP) to people at high risk of HIV infection.

1982   **NHS Reorganisation** – the area tier of NHS management is abolished resulting in the creation of 192 district health authorities (DHAs) that are responsible to the regional health authorities with the aim of simplifying the structure. This is the start of many more re-organisations over the next 3 decades **National Confidential Enquiry into Patient Outcome and Death (NCEPOD)** is born. A review of surgical and anaesthetic practice is reviewed over a year in 1982, known as the Confidential Enquiry into Peri-Operative Deaths (CEPOD). The venture is given government funding and renamed NCEPOD in 1988, extending its remit to include medical patients in 2002. Today, NCEPOD is an independent charity that reviews patient care by undertaking confidential surveys and research. NCEPOD reports have shaped the way healthcare is delivered in the UK, and their recommendations have created good practices such as peer review of mortality after surgery and ensuring hospitals admitting emergency patients have access to 24-hour radiology, operating and recovery rooms.

1983   **The Mental Health Act** introduces the issue of consent to treatment. Prior to this, a detained patient could be treated against their will, even if they were a 'voluntary' patient. The Mental Health Act allows people to be detained (or 'sectioned') against their will for the urgent treatment of mental disorders if they are at risk of harm to themselves or others.

The Griffiths Report is published, heralding a new managerial age in the NHS. It advocates NHS management boards at arm's length from the Government, and general managers with responsibility for performance and budgets in hospitals and district health authorities; bringing their experiences of business school and the private sector to NHS leadership. Doctors are encouraged to become involved with corporate decision making.

The UKCC (United Kingdom Central Council for Nursing, Midwifery and Health Visiting) is set up to replace the General Nursing Council in maintaining a register of nurses.

1986   **First case of BSE in cattle** is reported by the State Veterinary Service in the UK. Bovine Spongiform Encephalopathy or 'Mad Cow Disease' caused fatal changes to the brains of cows. In 1990, a domestic cat was diagnosed with the disease, raising concerns that transmission to humans was possible. Up until 1996, when the link is acknowledged, the Government told the public there was no evidence the disease could be passed onto humans. An estimated 400,000 cattle infected with BSE entered the food chain in the 1980s, and over the next 25 years, 177 people contracted and died from a disease with similar neurological symptoms called new variant Creutzfeldt-Jakob disease (vCJD) thought to be from eating contaminated beef. Mass slaughter of infected herds takes place and a ban on exporting British Beef is imposed by the European Union. The BSE enquiry is published in 2000 and concludes that the crisis was a result of intensive farming and cows being fed with dead animal remains. The Government's reassurance campaign was branded a mistake which left the public feeling betrayed.
Chernobyl nuclear disaster

1987   **Promoting Better Health** – The government's plans for improving health are published in this White Paper, pledging a fee for primary care doctors taking part in health promotion work such as health checks and immunisations. These proposals formed the basis of the 1990 GP contracts.

The world's first heart, liver and lung transplant takes place in Cambridge at Papworth hospital, carried out by Professor Sir Roy Calne and Professor John Wallwork. The patient survives ten years and her healthy heart is then donated to another transplant patient.

1988   **National cervical screening** introduced. Screening is the process of identifying individuals who appear healthy but may be at increased risk of a condition. It is an imperfect process and in every screen, there can be false positive and false negative results. Cervical screening aims to prevent cervical cancer by detecting and treating abnormalities of the cervix. Today, Liquid based cytology (LBC) is used to collect samples of cells from the cervix. Currently in England it is available to women aged between 25-64 years. Human Papilloma virus (HPV) is a common virus transmitted usually through sexual contact, which will be cleared by the immune system in the same way it would fight the common cold. There are over a 100 subtypes of this virus, and some high risk subtypes (HR-HPV) have been linked with the development of abnormal cervical cells – which left untreated, may go on to develop into cervical cancer. If cell changes are detected and HR-HPV is present, then women will be referred for colposcopy, where the cervix can be viewed under a microscope to determine if further treatment is required.

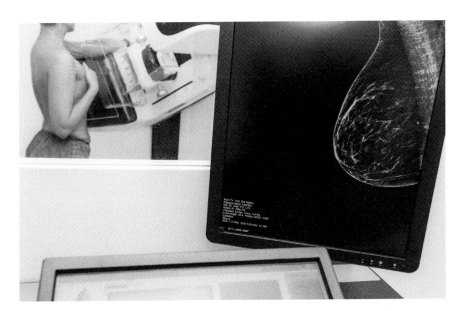

A mammogram (Abobe Stock Images)

Measles, mumps, rubella (MMR) vaccine introduced

Breast screening introduced. The Forrest Report on breast cancer screening concludes there was a convincing case to screen women over the age of 50 with mammograms (x-rays of the breasts), as long as there are effective resources in place to deal with any abnormalities found through the process.

Routine newborn hearing testing is introduced at Whipps Cross University Hospital using otoacoustic emission technology.

Lockerbie bombing

1989 **Working for Patients** – the Government's White Paper sets out plans to reform the NHS, introducing the creation of an internal market by splitting the bodies that provide care from those that purchase it. Health authorities are required to manage their own budgets to purchase the best possible healthcare services for their areas – even if that means favouring external organisations over their own local hospitals. Meanwhile, hospitals can apply to become NHS trusts – independent organisations with their own management. GPs with registered populations of at least 11,000 patients, are able to apply for practice budgets to purchase hospital services (known as 'Fundholding GPs').

Project 2000 is implemented following the Judge Report of 1985, which recommended the transfer of nurse training to Universities. Concerns are raised regarding acquisition of practical as well as academic skills.

Fall of the Berlin Wall

My NHS Story

Dr David Wingfield is a GP and senior partner at Brook Green Medical Centre in Hammersmith, and chairman of the Hammersmith and Fulham GP Federation. He reflects on his 30 years working in the NHS.

'As with many doctors, I suppose, I took my decision to specialise, in General Practice, because of the inspiration of another. My teacher David El Kabir demonstrated personal commitment to the people of Notting Hill building up his registered patient list from nothing and in doing so generated huge mutual commitment, the foundation of the relationship between doctor and patient.

'He inspired us, as his students, to found a charity for the homeless of central London, Wytham Hall, where we could care for them when sick and unable to endure the terrible hardships of life on the street. I entered the world of General Practice therefore assuming that a career founded on a vocation and public service was at the heart of the NHS. What a surprise was in store.

'One of my first awakenings was a conference on Single Homelessness in London where a report was launched and purported to offer solutions to an age-old problem. It was nothing of the kind. Whilst the SHIL report offered numerical analysis and quantities it had no depth of understanding. It asked for political shift but the direction was unclear because its whole analysis was superficial. While this report is now long confined to the history books, the cycle of reports offering analysis, understanding and solutions has continued unabated.

'The GP was always the poor relation of doctors in the NHS's 'hierarchy of specialties'. Competition between doctors to the point of aggression was commonplace and horrified many of us who had to endure consultants behaving like demigods. I wondered why this was this tolerated in a National Health Service that was supposed to deliver care to all patients equally and from cradle to grave The focus on the patient and holistic practice was it seemed to me understood to be a matter for the Nursing profession and the GP. After the foundation of the Royal College of GPs in 1952 these principles were enshrined in statute and seemed at least for a while to assure the foundations and purpose of the field I was committed to work within.

'When I was starting out as a GP it was thought that the NHS could be run more professionally and efficiently if a professional managerial element was introduced. The influential Griffiths Report (1983) ushered in this imaginative new dynamic era. But as Brian Jarman subsequently lamented in a BMJ editorial some 30 years later, managers remained in a fundamentally different place from clinical leaders and rather than complementing clinical leadership, management tried over time to control it. This has contributed to the current state whereby doctors at all levels of the NHS are disillusioned and confused by perceived controls over their clinical autonomy. Clinical leadership is now being reinvented, albeit in a straitjacket of guidelines and policies.

'Looking back over a career of over 30 years I see that key elements of the NHS have struggled to change.

'Firstly, there is a misunderstanding of what is required when confronted with a balance of risk. A limited analysis has too often been coupled with the reversion to bureaucracy and appeal to hierarchy when confronting difficult problems. "It was someone else's decision". "I had no ability to control or take the decision". I often now ask who is in charge only to find that no-one is able to answer. Consider, as an example the programme of planned hospital closures in North West London. There is no evidence that fewer hospital beds will be achievable; and even less that there is a systematic programme of replacement with community resources. Central London Hospitals on Red Alert with no beds is now sadly commonplace, even in summer.

'Secondly, there is an undue emphasis on a Public Health or the "population" viewpoint. Even though this has merit, it undermines the very personal relationship between the doctor and the patient. What is good for the many is not necessarily right for the individual. The widespread and increasing use of statin medication is a case in point. Many patients stand to gain from such treatment and the scientific basis is strong. But prescribing based on target populations and control of cholesterol levels to change outcomes for society is wrong at the an individual level. The patient may wish to make a different and more personal decision.

'The beginnings of professional accountability are emerging in the form of integrated services across primary and secondary care, hospital and community services, nurses and doctors. GPs nationwide are hearing the call to arms and forming organisations that offer the possibility of primary care services at scale (whether through large partnerships or federations of various forms). They may yet prove that the large scale GP in the NHS has a future. But shackled with senseless financial rules and contractual procedures (often distanced from outcomes) from an unaccountable managerial system makes me recall William Blake who wrote: "Bound and weary I thought best, to sulk upon my mother's breast".

'I look forward to an NHS which continues to deliver its founding principles, but I am not optimistic. The cracks are already emerging in the form of short-term solutions, outsourced services with poor contractual managerial control, and worst of all a financing system which is set on affordability rather than regard to the expectations of the service it delivers. NHS professional management has now had over 20 years to prove itself. It has not done so and should be reformed along with a return to a patient focused professionally led NHS with doctors playing a prominent part. Our patients (and I count myself in their number) will not forgive us if we let them down.'

1990s

The nineties saw increasing choices for patients and the creation of telephone services such as NHS Direct. Advances in technology and the rise of the internet shaped society, leading to the emergence of expert patients and multiple health charities. The Human Genome Project took off and gene therapy developed, as did cloning and the use of human tissue in medicine; whilst the MMR Scandal and GP serial killer Harold Shipman hit the headlines. The concept of Commissioning was introduced to the NHS in the early 1990s, when the 'internal market' was born – internal, because both buyers and sellers of services were NHS organisations. Commissioning is the process of planning, securing and monitoring services and until 1989, health authorities decided on the amount of care needed and provided it through their own hospitals. The Conservative government introduced these market theories into healthcare, on the premise that the public sector is inefficient, and the private sector brings growth and innovation. They argued that by making providers compete for resources, greater efficiency and innovation would be encouraged. When the Labour Party came into power in 1997, they fiercely opposed the internal market, and abolished GP Fundholding ... only to reverse their position and re-introduce it under a new name a few years later (Practice Based Commissioning). Labour also devolved power to an elected parliament in Scotland and an elected assembly in Wales and Northern Ireland, resulting in four separate health systems.

1990   **NHS reorganisation – The National Health Service Community Care Act** receives Royal assent, pushing through the proposals of the 1989 Working for Patients White paper to split the provision and purchasing (or commissioning) of healthcare. The act allowed the Secretary of State for Health to establish

NHS trusts by order. The trusts assumed responsibility for the ownership and management of hospitals that were previously managed by the regional or district health authorities.

New GP contracts for GPs saw greater external management of General Practice and established financial incentives for GPs to become more involved in health promotion activity. GPs received payment for collating information such as the height, weight and blood pressure of patients. The GP Fundholding system allowed GPs to take on responsibilities for commissioning services for patients, becoming more involved with the wider health system. Not all GPs become fundholders, and those who do not have services purchased for them by the local health authorities. This brings criticism that a two-tier system has been created, in which patients in practices with GP Fundholders are able to access care more rapidly.

The NHS Confederation is founded (initially as the National Association of Health Authorities and Trusts) as a membership body for NHS organisations. Members include acute and foundation trusts, community health service providers, mental health service providers, ambulance trusts and clinical commissioning groups. It claims to represent the whole NHS and runs an annual conference for senior decision makers.

Poll tax riots.

1991 **The Patients' Charter** is first published, setting out patients' rights within the NHS and the service they can expect to receive. The charter sets out targets for waiting times for hospital treatment

The Gulf War.

1992 **The Health of the Nation** White Paper is published and identifies coronary heart disease, cancer, mental health, HIV care, sexual health and accidents as areas for improvement. There is an emphasis on individual responsibility for health.

The Internet starts to take off in the UK as dial up internet access is introduced.

1994 **The NHS Organ Donor Register** is set up following a campaign by parents John and Rosemary Cox, whose son Peter died of a brain tumour and wanted to donate his organs to help others.

Patient's waiting for care (Adobe Stock Images)

NHS Reorganisation – the number of regional health authorities is reduced from fourteen to eight
The Channel Tunnel opens

1996   National Screening Committee established.

1997   **Labour government.**
The New NHS: Modern, Dependable is a White Paper produced by the new Labour government which leads to further NHS reorganisation. It aims to replace the internal market with a more integrated system, but still retains the purchaser-provider split introduced by the Conservatives. GP Fundholding is abolished due to concerns of a two-tier system.
Dolly the sheep – is born first mammalian clone

1998   **MMR Scandal begins** with the publication of a paper by Dr Andrew Wakefield in the The *Lancet* suggesting a link between the MMR (Measles, Mumps, Rubella) vaccination and autism. Parents across the world avoid vaccinating their children due to a fear of autism. Measles outbreaks and deaths in 2008 and 2009 are attributed to not vaccinating. Scientists published many more studies proving no link. Wakefield is investigated and found to be guilty of deliberate fraud and is struck off (removed from) the medical register. His study was funded by anti-vaccine lawyers and found to be full of ethical violations. He picked data that supported his argument and ignored data that didn't, and he deliberately falsified facts for financial gain. *The Lancet* subsequently withdrew his paper.

The National Institute for Clinical Excellence (NICE) and the Commission for Health Improvement is established as a special health authority to provide national guidance on quality and reduce variation in the availability and quality of NHS treatments – the so-called postcode lottery. NICE is responsible for producing national evidence-based guidance on health promotion, health technologies, social care and disease treatment and prevention. They also develop quality standards for those providing and commissioning services. (NICE is also responsible for developing QOF – the Quality Outcomes Framework – a voluntary incentive scheme for all GP practices in the UK, which rewards them financially

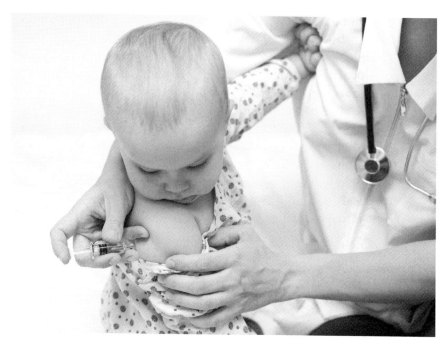

(Adobe Stock Images)

for how well they care for patients. Under the scheme, GP practices score QOF points (more about this later) according to their level of achievement against a series of indicators, such as the percentage of patients with a new diagnosis of a disease who are referred for certain tests. As part of the Health and Social Care Act 2012, NICE became established in legislation as a Non-Departmental Public Body (NDPB) accountable to the Department of Health, but operationally independent. NICE now attempts to assess the cost effectiveness of NHS expenditures to determine whether or not they represent value for money. New treatments are analysed relative to the next best treatment currently in use using Quality-Adjusted Life Years (QALY) to quantify the expected health benefits.

NHS Direct is set up as a 24 hour telephone advice line staffed by nurses, aiming to provide people with fast advice and information about health and NHS services at home. This closed in 2014 due to financial problems and was replaced by NHS 111, an 'urgent but not life threatening' advice line staffed by telephone operators, to complement the long running 999 emergency number. 999 is the world's oldest emergency telephone number and was introduced to London in 1937 after a house fire killed five women. An outraged neighbour complained she had been kept on hold when trying to contact the local fire brigade, and 999 was born.

The European Working Time Directive (EWTD) takes effect in UK law in October 1998 to protect the health and safety of workers in the European Union. It dictates minimum requirements regarding working hours, annual leave and rest periods. Doctors in training were exempt from the EWTD until August 2004. Its implementation was examined in a report commissioned by Medical Education England (now Health Education England) which found it had impacted training opportunities.

1999 **NHS Reorganisation.** After the abolition of GP Fundholding, 481 Primary Care Groups are created to replace it – technically subcommittees of the District Health Authorities. These later become Primary Care Trusts in 2000. A *BMJ* editorial comments that this reorganisation is 'universalising fundholding, while repudiating the concept'.
The Euro is introduced.

My NHS Story

Lianna Brinded is a Journalist and Broadcaster who shares her view that the NHS is broken and needs fixing now.

'The NHS is the jewel in the crown for Britain. Whoever you are, wherever you are, you can count on having a doctor or a nurse see to you for free. Well, when we mean free, funded by the taxpayer. Countries like the US have such a chronically expensive, complicated, and discriminatory system that if you're poor, you have to really weigh up whether you are able to afford those stitches because you fell over in the street, have that baby, or even potentially life-saving medication for your long-term illness. So, in comparison, the NHS looks like a dream.

'But this is a dangerous way of thinking. The NHS was probably fit for purpose 60 years ago but our society is larger, more diverse, and complex and the model that once was the saviour for the masses can now be an active hindrance for care.

'Our social media feeds are awash of people being grateful for the treatment they did or didn't have. It's full of stories of not being seen on time, being denied scans or treatment, or being told we're wasting NHS time. But you still have people peddling out this "but at least we have the NHS."

'The issue is that we are a nation of reactionary medicine and care, not preventative. The whole system runs on trying to fix things when it's too late rather than do the necessary scans, treatment, or care in the first place that would prevent long-term problems, pain, heartache, and death. When the NHS screws up, people are in pain, their livelihoods ruined, or even die.

'My family, like many others, is littered with stories of NHS horrors. My father, a previously healthy person, suddenly blacked out and had a fit. The hospital just said he was stressed and refused to give him even one scan. Turns out a year later he had a brain tumour sitting on his optic nerve that had grown rapidly in that one year. What happened next was a year of systematic bad care, mistakes, and corner cutting that helped accelerate his death. He wasn't even 50.

'My mother had a mild stroke in the middle of a restaurant that was conveniently located next door to one of London's top hospitals. The paramedics came and didn't take her across the road for treatment.

I urged and begged for her to get seen to—they wouldn't budge. The whole episode was even more distressing considering this is how my father was allowed to incubate a tumour that could've been dealt with had the doctors and other staff done the logical thing and requested scans. It's even more sickening that my Mum was a NHS nurse for decades and she couldn't even get the care when she needed it.

'Friends who have broken their legs, wrists, ankles, have been taken to hospital only to not even be given scans or treatment. Many have been left with problems that have resulted in corrective surgery years down the line or life-long mobility issues because they didn't get the right care in the first place. I know people who were incapable of breathing properly and diagnosed with asthma because it was easy to do so, in lieu of doing any investigations—turns out they were being strangled from the inside by abnormal growths.

'These tales aren't just isolated horror stories, they are part and parcel of the system we have today. But we can't blame the Government of not spending money—it's risen every year. It's about how the NHS uses it, which is a responsibility for the sector as well as people who use it.

'We have some of the worst hospital bed availability, we waste over £1 billion a year in missed appointments—and nearly the same amount has been wasted on a failed IT system. We quibble over giving an expensive scan to someone in the early stage of a disease, yet spend thousands more per person to fix something that could've been prevented. We have some of the worst cancer survival rates in Europe and parts of the developed world because we hold back on using certain drugs or giving the relevant treatment in the first place. There are campaigns telling us not to go to doctors for various things, even though that cough could be something sinister and could end up being an ailment that could kill the very young, old, or vulnerable.

'It's not just a structural change that's needed—it's an attitude change. For a "free" service, of course it will always feel under-funded, under-staffed. But then would everyone be willing to pay more out of their taxes? Tax hikes are deeply unpopular.

'Changing the NHS to a prevention service from a reactionary one will be hard but it's something that former health secretaries, doctors, and key NHS officials have been asking for. Not only will it make the whole system more efficient, it will also mean we use the money in the right way to give the care and treatment we all deserve.'

2000s

The new millennium brings with it further NHS reshuffling and financial crises. New Labour's victory in 1997 brought in the NHS Plan in 2000 which promised to rebuild the NHS for the twenty-first century. PFIs, PCTS and foundation trusts are born and the four hour target is introduced to emergency departments. Terrorism shocks the world with attacks in New York, Spain and closer to home in London. There is an influx of migrants, particularly from the European Union and retired Brits also emigrate to sunnier climes in their thousands, prompting the government to say that the NHS should not be free for those who do not live in the UK. Smoking is banned in public places in 2007 and smart phones and social media becomes normal by the end of the decade. The NHS tries to keep up by introducing the National Programme for IT, aiming for a paperless NHS. Its ultimate failure is deemed to be a result of an underestimation of the scale of the project, combined with a top down management approach – including centralised authorities making decisions on behalf of local organisations, with a lack of adequate engagement with the people actually using it.

2000   **The NHS Plan** sets out a strategy to increase staffing, hospital beds and decrease waiting times. This is formalized by the 2001 Health and Social Care Act. A new model of financing is agreed called the **Private Finance Initiative (PFI),** which involves using private sector money instead of public money. Loans are taken from private companies with high interest rates (some over 70 per cent per cent) to build new hospitals and clinics, which the NHS is required to pay off like a mortgage over the following decades. These schemes are poorly negotiated by civil servants against opportunistic financiers resulting in huge debts for NHS trusts. A report from the Centre for Health and the Public interest in 2017 showed that companies running PFI contracts between 2010-2015, to build and run NHS hospitals and services made pre-tax profits of £831million from the NHS. This money has been taken away from patient care and is often more than it cost to build the hospitals in the first place. Over the next five years, £1billion of taxpayers funds will go towards paying for PFIs.

NHS Walk in Centres open to deal with minor illnesses and injuries offering round the clock access. They are nurse led and available to everyone without needing an appointment or needing to register.

2001 **Bristol Heart Scandal** report published. During the 1990s, high mortality rates were found among babies undergoing cardiac surgery at the Bristol Royal Infirmary. The inquiry revealed a lax approach to safety, with a lack of leadership, teamwork and staff shortages, which ultimately led to the development of regulatory bodies (see below).
The Commission for Healthcare Improvement is created, as directed by the Health Act of 1999. This is the first organization to formally assess the performance of NHS hospitals (now known as the Care Quality Commission or CQC)
The National Patient Safety Agency is set up (now part of NHS Improvement) to drive improved patient care, prompted by reports such as the DoH's report 'An Organization with a Memory'. This suggested that every year, 28,000 written complaints are made about aspects of clinical treatment in NHS hospitals; that hospital-acquired infections cost the NHS £1billion and that over £400million is paid by the NHS annually to settle clinical negligence claims.
9-11 Terrorist Attack on the World Trade centre

2002 **NHS Reorganisations.** Based on the White Paper 'Shifting the Balance of Power', 95 Health authorities are abolished and partly replaced by **Primary Care Trusts (PCTs)** which are set up as administrative bodies, responsible for commissioning healthcare, and 28 strategic health authorities, which are to provide regional management for the NHS and oversee the PCTs. The PCTs are given responsibility for 80 per cent per cent of the health budget.
The Nursing and Midwifery Council (NMC) is founded to regulate nurses and midwives and set educational standards, replacing the UKCC.
National Programme for IT (NPfIT)is launched with the idea of creating a paperless NHS, with an integrated IT system throughout the entire NHS (30,000 GPs and 300 hospitals). An agency called NHS Connecting for Health was formed in

2005 to deliver this project (replacing what was before it – the NHS Information Authority). The motivation for the ambitious project came from Cabinet level, but the delivery did not translate into reality. Hit by technical problems and contractual wrangling, the £11bn scheme was scrapped in 2011 and labelled a fiasco. The Health and Social Care Information centre (HSCIC) was created as a special health authority and took over parts of the NPfIT in 2013 when NHS Connecting for Health ceased to exist. It was rebranded as the catchier NHS Digital in 2016. NHS Digital now runs the Spine service in England – a central, secure system for patient data. This comprises the Electronic Prescription service, which sends prescriptions digitally from GPs to pharmacies; The Summary Care Record-which allows authorized NHS staff to see important clinical information about patients to provide the best care; the E-referral Service which manages the booking of hospital appointments; the Child Protection Information Sharing Service which helps collate safeguarding concerns.

The Wanless Report, commissioned by the Treasury to look at healthcare spending and future trends, concluded that future NHS spending would rise, mainly due to patients demanding more choice and higher quality services. The author recommended spending more on IT and enhancing the role of primary care.

2003   **NHS Reorganisation**. The Health and Social care (Community Standards) Act is passed, allowing for the establishment of foundation trusts and new GP contracts. This act introduced 'Alternate Provider Medical Services' or APMS contracts, which allowed non-NHS providers to be commissioned by the PCTs to deliver care.

Foundation Trusts are established as part of the government's plan to continue the internal market. There are set up as a 'halfway house' between the public and private sectors to try to make healthcare more efficient. Foundation status aims to give trust managers financial and managerial freedom from the Department of Health, by allowing them to borrow money privately, without prior approval from the Treasury, and invest this money as they see fit in local services

Monitor is established to regulate NHS foundation trusts in terms of quality and finances. It became part of NHS Improvement in 2016

Independent Sector Treatment Centres (ISTC) are first opened. These centers focus on providing routine elective treatments, (such as cataract surgery) for NHS patients by the private sector as part of the 2000 NHS Plan to reduce NHS waiting lists, promising greater efficiency and patient choice. They promised more than they delivered. Unable to employ NHS staff at the outset, they were staffed by overseas doctors, whose quality of training and familiarity with the NHS was questioned. They negatively impacted the training of junior doctors, who previously learned by doing the 'straightforward' procedures the ISTCs took on. The finances were also problematic, in that they were paid whether they reached the required targets or not. They were not regulated in the same way as the NHS, and data could not be collected on their productivity in the same way as in the NHS due to commercial sensitivity and poor data collection.

Tobacco Adverts banned Severe acute respiratory syndrome (SARS) global outbreak

2004   **New GP Contracts** are renegotiated, resulting in more autonomy for practices regarding the range of services they provide and a focus on performance related pay for reaching standards set out in the Quality and Outcomes Framework (QOF). Stronger regulatory mechanisms are introduced for GPs including annual appraisals and a requirement to register with the CQC. GPs traditionally carried out evening house calls and emergency night visits providing continuity to their patients, either individually, or as part of a GP co-operative. The new contracts allowed GPs to opt out of this (virtually all did) passing responsibility for out of hours care to the PCTs. Social-enterprises replaced most of the co-operatives (non-for-profit-organisations) and private companies (such as Harmoni, Serco and Virgin) stepped in to plug the gaps costing more than £392 million in 2005. Hospital consultant's contracts are also re-negotiated, aiming to increase the direct amount of time they spend with patients.

Four Hour Targets are introduced into emergency departments to reduce waiting times. The NHS Plan in 2000 stated that by 2004, no-one should be waiting for more than four hours in the emergency department from arrival to admission, transfer or discharge, and financial incentives to meet these targets were introduced. Government funding was invested in recruiting new ED nurses increasing consultant numbers. New strategies were introduced to achieve these targets and improve patient flow. Emergency Nurse Practitioners (ENPs) assessed and treated patients with minor injuries to avoid the wait to see a doctor, and money was invested in other NHS services – such as NHS Direct and GP out of hours care. Waiting times did reduce, however reports of compromised patient care due to management pressures to meet the targets were notably reported in the Mid Staffs enquiry. Targets are a way for the Government to focus the entire NHS on a priority, which they can then show to voters and taxpayers to explain what their money is achieving.

Agenda for Change (AfC) comes into operation, and remains the grading and pay system used for staff in the NHS (with the exception of doctors, dentists and some managers). It allocates posts to set paybands to try to evaluate the job rather than the person doing it, to create uniformity across the NHS.

Facebook launched.

Boxing Day Tsunami An earthquake in the Indian Ocean on Boxing Day is the third largest earthquake ever recorded triggering a series of tsunamis throughout Asia. It is one of the deadliest natural disasters in recorded history.

2005   **The Shipman Inquiry is closed.** GP and serial killer Harold Shipman shattered the faith in the medical profession after he was exposed as a serial killer, responsible for the deaths of up to 215 patients. The inquiry started after his trial in 2000, with the final report being release in 2005. Shipman was jailed for life for murdering fifteen of his patients, and subsequently committed suicide in jail. An array of changes were introduced following the inquiry, including changes to the death certification process, safer management of controlled drugs and monitoring of prescribing data, systems to monitor mortality rates and unexpected deaths, revalidation and appraisal of GPs and GP practice inspections.

London Terrorist Bombings

Modernising Medical Careers (MMC) replaced the traditional training grades in postgraduate medical education. The traditional first year Pre-Registration House Officer (PRHO) and first year Senior House Officer (SHO) grades were replaced by a 2 year Foundation Programme (Foundation House Officer 1 and 2, or F1 and F2). Further speciality training replaced the old Specialist Registrar (SpR) grade, with trainees being awarded a certificate of completion of training (CCT) and entry to the specialist or GP register at the end of training. MMC was part of the NHS Plan 2000 which aimed to increase consultant numbers by 'modernising the SHO grade' or reducing the amount of training time doctors undertake before they become consultants. The old system allowed doctors the flexibility to try a variety of different jobs and gain valuable experience before deciding what to specialise in. The transition to the new system was disastrous. The Postgraduate Medical Education and Training Board initially recruited centrally, resulting in thousands of doctors being left without jobs, followed by apologies from the Health Secretary Patricia Hewitt and a judicial review of the system.

2006 **NHS Bowel Screening Programme** is launched, offering home faecal occult blood testing, detecting an estimated 3,000 cancers each year

Bilingual no smoking signs 2007
(Science Museum, London)

2007 **Smoking is banned** in restaurants, pubs and public places in England. A year after this, there is a significant decline in hospital admissions for heart attacks, asthma and lung infections.

Iphone launched.

2008 **HPV (Human papilloma virus) vaccination programme** is launched to help prevent cervical cancer.

GP training – The RCGP publish a training curriculum for GPs and completion of the assessments for the postgraduate Membership of the Royal College of General Practitioners (MRCGP) becomes compulsory. This is equivalent to the postgraduate qualifications of MRCP and FRCS that are required to become a hospital physician or surgeon respectively.

The Darzi Review – High Quality Care for All is published led by Lord Ara Darzi, a colorectal surgeon and Minister. A year long review of the NHS is carried out, engaging 65,000 healthcare staff, patients and the public to discuss visions for the future of the NHS, and to examine barriers to delivering these visions.

Global Financial Crisis.

2009 **The NHS Constitution** is published, setting out the rights and responsibilities of patients, staff and trust boards and the guiding principles which govern the service

The NHS Abdominal Aortic Aneurysm (AAA) Screening Programme is launched, aimed at detecting and treating large aneurysms early before they (often fatally) rupture. The screening programme invites men over the age of 65 to have an abdominal ultrasound scan to detect enlargement of the main blood vessel in the abdomen. This is not offered to women, as evidence suggests they are less likely to develop aneurysms than men, therefore screening can do more harm than good.

Swine Flu Epidemic

Barack Obama becomes the first African American President of the USA

My NHS Story

Hannah Ramsdale is a nurse on the neurosciences ward at the John Radcliffe Hospital in Oxford. She shares her experiences of the NHS.

'I qualified as an Adult Nurse (DipHE) in the summer of 2005. During my last few placements, in my third year of training, "Agenda for Change" was being implemented, to review and change nurses' pay structure and banding. I understood that upon qualifying I would become a Band 5 Staff Nurse and no longer a D Grade Staff Nurse. I can remember discussing it with my mentors and other nurses at the time and being incredulous about a question they were being asked in a survey about the changes: "Are you ever interrupted whilst trying to complete a task?" The exasperation, shock, irritation and laughter – as sometimes it's the only thing to do – I remember was from the nurses (who would become my colleagues), who knew, before I really did, that the answer was... yes. Persistently. Of course, we are.

During every task, job, patient wash, dressing, drug round, handover, phone call, ward round, patient conversation, you are pulled and pushed in a variety of different directions: to a deteriorating patient, a colleague, urgent post-operative observations, doctor's instructions. I must also add that I became a nurse straight after completing my A levels. I have never known or worked in a corporate or business environment. This is all I know. I have now worked in the NHS for over a decade. I suspect most nurses may find my career path a bit backwards: most would have started out on the wards. However, once qualified I became a Band 5 Anaesthetic and Recovery nurse for Plastic and Neuro surgery. This lead me in less than a year to get a Staff Nurse position in Neuro Intensive Care (NICU), were I worked for four years. During this time, I travelled to Australia and worked as a Staff Nurse on a Medical Ward in Queensland. After leaving NICU in 2010 I held a brief community nurse role which then lead me back to the Neurosciences Ward, working with and caring for surgical patients, where I have worked for the last five years.

'I think in recent years, my experience of the NHS and especially in the ward I work, is that it is in constant motion. No sooner has a bed space has been cleaned and the bed made, another patient or even two, are already waiting for it. I'm not sure it is possible to move fast enough anymore. I find it extremely frustrating how much each department works separately to the next – in terms of respecting the enormity of each other's jobs and roles. We are all striving for the same thing. An absurd hierarchy of 'busy-ness' is maintained by all. The NHS isn't busy. It is overwhelmed. I'm not sure there is an accurate word to describe the environment, the system. People's lives are altered – and lost. Since I have been working in the NHS, I feel the patient's expectations of it are far too high. They over-estimate what it is and what can be achieved. Yes, it has achieved such an incredible amount, and the public need that to be true for their mum, dad, auntie, uncle, brother and sister. But when it isn't and either small things happen, or catastrophic events occur, blame must be placed and owned by someone. That is human nature. Though human nature is what makes every NHS Trust exist around the country. And it is human nature that drives every staff member from our cleaning and clerical staff to Consultants and Directors and everyone in between.

'A keen interest of mine, that I've spent time highlighting on the ward is dignity and privacy. I found out about Dignity Champions in 2011, (run by the National Dignity Council) and have been holding Dignity Day events (held nationally on 1st February) on the ward each year. To find out from patients and relatives what we are doing well and those areas that need improvement. The smallest change can take the longest time to implement even with assistance of senior ward management. It is always the little things that make a huge difference. I strive to do those small things as well as looking after my clinical caseload. Washing a lady's hair having waited a week after surgery. Cleaning a patient's glasses. Helping a patient wash their hands before lunch. Brushing someone's teeth. Combing their hair. Putting on their favourite perfume/aftershave. It matters. I find my job a privilege. To care for someone at their most vulnerable is a privilege. The NHS horror stories that fill our news and conversations are real. Though I could provide the same number or more of wonder stories. Patients' lives that I'm unlikely to ever forget.

'What I think now though, is that I won't be a nurse till I retire. I am not quite ready to give up my registration just yet, but I honestly can't sustain the pressure of this environment. So very regrettably I can see that my skills need to be directed into a different area and role.'

2010s

The 2010s brought a series of NHS bad news stories – the Francis report, budget deficits, patient dissatisfaction and emergency services in crisis. Increasing healthcare costs were driven by the ageing population, expensive new treatments and increased expectations. Ongoing austerity measures, pay freezes and imposed junior doctor contracts demoralized NHS staff, whose loyalty and goodwill notoriously kept the NHS afloat. This led to junior doctor strikes and an exodus of NHS staff overseas. Nonetheless, the public's affection for the NHS remained strong, and this was demonstrated and celebrated during the opening ceremony of the London 2012 Olympic Games. The passing of the Conservative Government's 2012 Health and Social Care Act was one of the biggest reforms the NHS has ever seen, argued by some to mark the end of the NHS – not only by encouraging privatisation and thus fragmentation, but by ending the duty of the Health Secretary to provide health services to the nation. The referendum on membership of the European Union lead to a Brexit vote, and the UK Independence Party (UKIP) grew in strength. As the decade closed, clusters of a mysterious pneumonia were being reported in a city called Wuhan in China. Little did we know as the New Year Eve fireworks welcomed in 2020, how the world was about to transform. Over seventy years on, the world is a different place to the post war era in which it was born, and the NHS is now way past retirement age, however, it is still standing. For how much longer, remains to be seen. The public of 1948, who stoically suffered through the Second World War are gone, and today we have a more atomised consumerist society, with a culture of instant gratification. Aneurin Bevan was famously asked how long the NHS would survive, and he replied 'As long as there are folk left with the faith to fight for it.'

2010   **Coalition Government (Conservative/Liberal Democrats)**

2011   **Arab Spring.**
Greek Financial Crisis
The NHS Constitution is published by the Department of Health, setting out the guiding principles of the organisation and the rights of NHS patients and staff. The NHS belongs to the people and the principles set by Bevan in 1948 remain core to the constitution, free at the point of delivery, meeting the

needs of everyone and based on clinical need, not the ability to pay. All NHS bodies and private and third sector providers to the NHS are obliged by law to take account of the constitution when making decisions. The constitution is renewed every ten years and any government that wishes to alter the principles and values of the NHS must first engage in a full and transparent debate with the public, patients and staff.

There are now seven key principles that guide the NHS:

- The NHS provides a comprehensive service to all
- Access to NHS services is based on clinical need, not an individual's ability to pay
- The NHS aspires to the highest standards of excellence and professionalism
- The NHS aspires to put patients at the heart of everything that it does
- The NHS works across organisational boundaries and in partnership with other organisations in the interest of patients, local communities and the wider population.
- The NHS is committed to providing best value for taxpayers' money and the most effective, fair and sustainable use of finite resources.
- The NHS is accountable to the public, communities and patients that it serves

UK riots following the death of Mark Duggan, a man shot dead by the police. Thousands of people rioted in London and other cities throughout the UK and the chaos this creates leads to looting, arson and 5 deaths. Racial tension and gang culture, combined with economic decline and unemployment are debated as the cause for the breakdown in social morality seen during the riots.

2012 **The Health and Social Care Act 2012** – is passed in April 2013, bringing some of the most extensive reforms the NHS has ever seen. Since Bevan held the position in 1948, the Secretary of State for Health had been held responsible for providing a national health service. But this Bill severed this duty and delegated it to CCGs (Clinical Commissioning Groups). PCTs (Primary Care Trusts) and SHAs (Strategic Health Authorities) are abolished and replaced by CCGs which were partly run by GPs but provided access for private providers as well. The Any Qualified Provider (AQP) scheme allows private companies to compete for NHS funded work. It essentially legislates for reductions in government funded health services, while being unclear about who is ultimately responsible for people's health services; creating new powers for charging and heralding a shift from tax funded healthcare to a one in which patients may have to pay.

Revalidation is implemented. All UK doctors are legally required to be revalidated every 5 years if they wish to retain their licence to practice. The process is based upon demonstrating up to date knowledge, by undertaking continuous professional development (CPD) and providing multisource feedback from patients and colleagues. The idea for revalidation was raised in the 1970s (The Merrison Report), but it was a series of high profile scandals (Shipman, Bristol Heart Scandal) that shaped the implementation of this process.

London 2012 Olympic Games – Danny Boyle pays tribute to the ethos of the NHS in his opening ceremony, celebrating free healthcare for all as a core value of British Society. The NHS was founded in 1948, but this was also the last time the Olympic Games had been held in London.

2013   **NHS England** forms to oversee the commissioning of NHS services in England and to set the priorities and direction of the NHS.

Public Health England is formed as a result of the reforms. Prior to 2013, public health operated through the PCTs (via the Department of Health's Health Protection Agency, and via the Strategic Health Authorities at a regional level). In April 2013, these responsibilities are returned to local authorities (where they had been up until the 1973 NHS reorganisations) and Public Health England is created as a distinct organisation with operational autonomy from the Government. The Department of Health restyles itself as a strategic director of both NHS England and Public Health England – meaning that the responsibilities to provide health care and public health services lies with these organisation, rather than with the Government themselves. In the context of COVID-19, these measures were disastarous. They removed and fragmented local services for communicable disease control, scattering specialist staff, reducing their numbers and effectiveness on the ground. Austerity measures led to cuts to local authorities (up to 49.1%) and PHE made 'savings' of £500million over five years in the name of efficiency.

NHS Trust Development Authority is formed to oversee the management and governance of NHS non-Foundation Trusts (managed by Monitor) Trusts

Healthwatch England is created as a statutory accountability body, as the latest reorganization to involve patients and the public in the running of the NHS. 152 local Healthwatch groups were established in each local authority area, and were allocated £43.5 million of the NHS budget to share ideas on how to improve health and social care services. Budgets have been cut each year, and their role has been criticized by the People's Inquiry into London's NHS, who believe the organization should be abolished.

The Francis Inquiry Report is published, a public inquiry chaired by Robert Francis QC, examining the failings in care at the Mid-Staffordshire NHS Foundation trust between 2005-2009 – initiated due to its high mortality rates. Whole system failures are highlighted: insufficient and inexperienced staff with insufficient training and a lack of beds and resources. Relatives speak of family members being left in pain, unwashed and without access to food, water or the toilet. In 2006, the trust was tasked with saving £10million, and to achieve this, 150 staff were sacked and over 100 beds were taken away, resulting in a hospital unable to function, leading to situations where good people can do bad things. The 'Hard Truths' response to the inquiry announced that finances and targets would never again come before quality of care and new safety schemes were proposed.

2014　**NHS ranked first** by the Commonwealth Fund in a comparison of ten healthcare systems across the world (Australia, Canada, France, Germany, Netherlands, New Zealand, Norway, Sweden, Switzerland and the USA). The NHS comes top in terms of efficiency, safe and effective care, co-ordinated care, patient centred care and cost. However the NHS ranked 10th (last) on keeping people alive, some say, the primary function of healthcare. This is based on a composite 'healthy lives' score, which includes deaths among infants and patients who would have survived had they received timely and effective healthcare.

The NHS Five Year Forward View is published, focusing on preventing patients getting ill and recognising the need for the NHS to adapt to our changing society. It sets out practical steps for the NHS to deliver a more joined up service based around new models of care, such as providing care traditionally delivered in a hospital (like chemotherapy) in people's own homes and working in new ways. For example asking dementia specialists to conduct their clinics in GP surgeries, to improve access for those who need it.

GPs increasingly start to federate

Ebola virus outbreak in West Africa.

Scotland votes to remain in the UK.

Marriage (Same Sex Couples) Act 2013 came into force and the first marriages take place in 2014.

2015   **Conservative Government.**

Sustainability and Transformation Plans (STPs) are introduced in NHS planning guidance as part of the Five Year Forward View to deal with the expected increase in demand for services coupled with the anticipated decrease in funding. They take a 'place based approach' focusing on NHS spending in named geographical areas across England; where leaders are asked to identify the key priorities for their local areas, and plan to improve efficiency of services by integrating with social care and local authority services, whilst delivering financial balance. NHS England describes STPs as collective discussion forums, which bring together organisations who have historically done their own thing. For example, the Lancashire and Cumbria STP brought together thirty-one different statutory bodies to discuss their area plans – nine CCGs, six NHS provider trusts, four local authorities and twelve district councils. Millions were spent engaging private management consultants in these plans.

Morecambe Bay Inquiry report published. Significant failures in care come to light at the maternity department at Furness General Hospital between 2004-2013, which may have contributed to the deaths of three mothers and sixteen babies. They find poor working relationships between midwives, obstetricians and paediatricians and a 'them and us' attitude which hampers communication. Clinical competence among some staff fell below the expected levels, and a failure to perform adequate risk assessments, with an 'over-zealous' pursuit of natural childbirth by some midwives, led to unsafe care. Recommendations are to correct these problems, with an emphasis on reviewing serious incidents and learning from them. A national review of maternity provision in rural, isolated and difficult to recruit areas is advised.

2016   **Junior Doctors' Strike.** At a time when health spending is at its lowest since the Second World War, the government decides to push forward their plans for a 'Seven Day NHS' to extend the availability of non-emergency clinical services throughout

Save the NHS demonstration. (via Wikimedia Commons)

(© Telegraph Media Group Limited)

the entire week – without providing the necessary planning, funding and staffing to do so. (It is worth highlighting here that emergency care is provided 24/7 already). The Morecambe Bay and Mid Staffs Scandals demonstrated what happens when a service is poorly staffed, prompting proclamations that such poor care should rightly never happen again, but then the underlying issues of unsafe staffing and resources appear to be forgotten as the Health Secretary, Jeremey Hunt, makes the decision to impose the contracts for his vote winning 'Seven Day NHS', without coherently planning how he was going to deliver it. BMA negotiations break down, leading to strikes. The conflict is spun as a pay dispute, and the press label junior doctors as 'selfish, infantile, self-deluding idiots', igniting the fury of ordinarily placid junior doctors across the land, who are fearful of the implications of the contract. Being paid less is obviously galling but stretching the already crumbling 5 day service over 7 days – without any extra doctors – would increase workforce strain, and ultimately reduce patient safety and quality of care. Weekend admission continues to have a 10% higher mortality rate than weekday admission for all types of illness and public opinion is torn between supporting hard working junior doctors, and frustration at an inconvenient system.

The Cities and Local Government Devolution Bill is passed, allowing Secretaries of State to remove powers and duties from public bodies such as NHS trusts and commissioners, and transfer them to local councils or city authorities. This raises concerns about just where accountability will lie in an increasingly devolved NHS.

NHS Improvement is launched to regulate all NHS providers as a merger of Monitor (which regulated NHS foundation trusts) and the Trust Development Authority (which regulated all other trusts).

Brexit – the UK votes to leave the European Union. The implications of this for the NHS remain to be seen but European migrants make up a significant proportion of the workforce and scrapping of regulations such as the EU Working Time Directive will result in further staffing issues.

Donald Trump elected as president of the USA.

2017   **Next steps on the NHS Five Year Forward View** published by NHS England describes how its focus is evolving from STPs to Integrated Care Systems (ICSs) – also known as Accountable Care Organisations (ACOs) or Accountable Care Systems (ACSs). These are population-based models of care inspired by US organisations, that integrate primary, secondary, community and other health services. The plan is for STPs to evolve into ACSs, in which commissioners, providers and local authorities join together to take collective responsibility for the health of their local area. Some areas may move towards ACOs, which are slightly different, in that commissioners in that area will hold a contract with a single organisation for the majority of health care provision. **Staffing issues** continue and the British Medical Association's annual representative meeting highlights significant gaps in doctor's rotas. Following a 2016 report from the Royal College of Physicians (where 80 per cent per cent of doctors reported harmful and unsustainable levels of excessive stress at work), it suggests this is causing low morale and ever growing workloads.

RCEM Vision 2020 Campaign. (Reproduced with permission from the Royal College of Emergency Medicine)

RCEM Vision 2020 Following the worst four-hour performance in Emergency Departments for fifteen years, The Royal College of Emergency Medicine makes a plan to fix the staffing, systems and support in Emergency departments. Since 2010/11, A&E attendances in England increased by 7.4 per cent per cent (equivalent to the workflow of ten medium-sized emergency departments); but the workforce and resources did not increase to meet this demand. More hospital beds and better integration of other services is called for to reduce pressure on A&E. Instead of spending £1.3million a day on locum staff (as is currently the case), the College also calls for increased consultant numbers and increased training posts.

The Lord Darzi Review of Health and Care Interim Report is published, a decade after his first report, to examine and reform the quality and funding of health and care services within the NHS. The full report is planned to be released on the NHS's seventieth birthday.

The Windrush Scandal. Hundreds of commonwealth citizens, many from the 'Windrush' generation are wrongly detained, deported and denied legal rights in the UK (see Box 3.1)

Box 3.1 The Windrush Scandal

The 'Windrush' generation describes those people who came to the UK from Caribbean countries between 1948-1973 - many to take jobs in the NHS and other sectors requiring labour following the UK's post war labour shortage. The name comes from the ship that brought the first travellers - the 'HMT Empire Windrush'. When they arrived to the shores of the UK, the Caribbean was part of the British Commonwealth, which meant these people were automatically British subjects, free to permanently live and work in the UK.

In 2012, the UK government announced a 'Hostile Environment' policy to enforce immigration controls. It required employers, banks, landlords and the NHS to make the UK impossible to navigate for undocumented migrants, with the aim to push them to leave.

Many of the Windrush generation arrived as children, travelling on their parents passports. The records of their landing had long been destroyed by the Home Office, which meant many of these people lacked the documentation they needed to prove their right to remain in the UK. The Home Office demanded proof of residency from every year they had lived in the UK prior to the seventies, creating an impossible burden for people who had done nothing wrong.

Labelled falsely as 'illeagal immigrants' they lost access to housing, healthcare, bank accounts and driving licences. Some were placed in immigration detention, while others were deported to countries they hadn't been to since they were children.

The Hostile Environment policy remains in place. In March 2020, a review was published explaining that the scandal was no accident, but a result of deliberate anti-immigration policy aimed at reducing non-white immigration from the Commonwealth. It destroyed the lives of many black and minority ethnic British people.

My NHS Story

Denise Tyrell worked as community midwife in Leeds before retirement. She travelled to the UK from the West Indies in 1958 as part of the 'Windrush Generation'. This is her NHS Story.

Prize giving Day - Denise Tyrell - Front left

'I left St. Kitts and Nevis when I was only 17, to join my husband in the UK. The journey across the Atlantic took 2 weeks. I travelled by 'banana boat' with my 9 month old little girl, sharing a berth with 3 others. I didn't know anyone, but my husband was there to meet me when I made it to the UK. I just remember feeling so cold when I arrived. It was August, and I had a coat but I was shivering!'

'We took the train up to Leeds (me and the baby – the train left without my husband who was trying to load our luggage!) and I eventually embarked on my nurse training at St. James' Hospital, (in what is now the Thackray Medical Museum) to become a State Enrolled Geriatric Nurse.'

'I wanted to continue my training in Leeds to become a State Registered Nurse, but they were not taking on coloured nurses at that point. That is just how it was in those days. They didn't like to take on married nurses either. I passed more exams and was accepted to train at Stepping Hill hospital in Stockport. I lived in nurse's accommodation and only saw my family at weekends for two and a half years.'

'After passing my final exams, I was accepted to do my midwifery training back in Leeds, and once qualified, I worked in the community, which I loved. I got to know people, and saw the babies grow into adults. There were more home births back then. We looked after mums and babies for longer too, now the care seems to stop after a few weeks, which doesn't give much support to new families, especially if they need help breastfeeding.'

'I spent a lot of time training up new student nurses. I always remember one white student joined me on a delivery and the patient assumed she was in charge because of her colour – and she didn't correct them. I let her get on with things, watching in the background, until she found herself stuck and had to turn and ask me for help. She didn't make that mistake again!

'When I was on call, I could be called out to any part of Leeds. The ambulance crew would call to give me directions. All I had was an A to Z and I always found my way. I have a sat nav these days and get lost more than I did back then! I'd ask the patient to leave their light on for me to make sure I had the right house.'

'I've been shielding for the last few months due to COVID-19. It's strange having to stay in the house. It never really bothered me before, but someone telling me I have to stay in makes me want to go out even more.'

(Oral History)

2018   **Hadiza Bawa-Garba** is struck off the GMC's medical register in January 2018 after being found guilty of manslaughter on the grounds of gross negligence in 2015. In 2011, 6-year-old Jack Adcock was admitted to the Children's Assessment Unit at the Leicester Royal Infirmary with diarrhoea, vomiting and difficulty in breathing. He had an underlying heart condition and Down's Syndrome, which made the sepsis he was suffering with difficult to detect. A series of significant errors were identified in his care and he died later that evening after going into cardiac arrest. Paediatric trainee Dr Bawa-Garba was the ST4 Specialist Registrar who treated him that day. She was alone, covering the Emergency Department and the Children's Assessment Unit, with no senior consultant available on site. Rota gaps meant she was covering the work of two other doctors as well as her own, assessing multiple sick patients and, if this wasn't stressful enough, an IT failure in the hospital delayed any test results being available. She had also just recently returned from maternity leave. She was criticised for not specifically asking her consultant to review Jack – although she did share his clearly abnormal blood results with him during the evening handover meeting, and the consultant did not review on his own initiative. She was also criticised for not making it clear to Jack's Mum that he should not receive his regular blood pressure mediation while he was unwell, and she deliberately did not prescribe this on Jack's drug chart. Tragically, Jack was given this medication, which, combined with the sepsis, led to circulatory shock and cardiac arrest. The case has raised debate about how medical errors are dealt with – particularly in this case, where system failures and the pressures of under-staffing all contributed to the death of a little boy. But other individual members of staff were singled out (Nurse Isabel Amaro was also struck off the Nursing Register for her involvement). Medics across the country spoke out at the verdict of this case, not to minimise or excuse the potentially avoidable death of a child – but recognising that the appalling working conditions Bawa-Garba was battling through that day allowed the negligence to happen. We all recognised, with fear and vulnerability that the same conditions are occurring across the NHS every day, and that any doctor could be in the same position. The GMC's management of the case is highly criticised. They appealed to the High Court when its own regulators (the MPTS) gave her what it considered too lenient a punishment (one year suspension). This led to her erasure from the medical register, a decision that has subsequently been reversed. The GMC made no attempt to investigate the chaos at the Leicester Royal Infirmary that day, or her 'supervising' consultant, who contributed to the poor care delivered to Jack Adcock.

Whistleblowing The case of Dr Chris Day is highlighted in view of the Bawa-Garba ruling. Junior doctor Chris Day raised concerns about under staffing in an Intensive Care Unit in London in 2013. Instead of tackling the patient safety issues raised, Health Education England (HEE) and the local NHS trust attempted to discredit Day and block his whistleblowing case being heard. GMC guidance clearly states that they will exercise statutory powers against doctors who do not take prompt action to deal with patient safety concerns. But when juniors do speak out there is no protection, and Day lost his career as a result. Whistleblowing doctors are marked as troublemakers in the management culture of the NHS, and the Francis Report identified this as a reason for the silence of many medical staff in Mid Staffs. Both Bawa-Garba and Day's cases highlight problems in the NHS culture in that you are 'damned if you do and damned if you don't'.

Sugar Cubes Campaign. (Used with permission from Public Health, Liverpool City Council)

The Sugar Tax is introduced in an attempt to reduce sugar consumption and tackle obesity. Manufacturers of soft drinks are obliged to pay a levy on the high-sugar drinks they sell. Drinks with more than 8g of sugar per 100ml will face a tax rate of 24p per litre. The treasury expects to raise £240 million per year, which will be invested in breakfast clubs and school sports.

NHS70 Seventy years of the NHS is celebrated across the UK. 'Opt-Out' organ donation. The Government announces the introduction of an 'opt-out' rather than 'opt-in' system for organ and tissue donation.

My NHS Story

Dr Alison Gill is a Consultant in Respiratory Medicine at York Teaching Hospital NHS Foundation Trust and shares her views on the NHS

'I joined the NHS in 2004, and have always found it both a pillar of UK life, and a perpetually-changing, ever more political machine. It is simultaneously an astonishingly successful system, and on occasion a lesson in inefficiency.

'House jobs were a fantastic year, with a busy but enjoyable job and amazing team spirit, combined with my first experience of true financial independence, and a great work/life balance. Mine was the last year before most hospitals transitioned to foundation programmes, and I was also one of the last to benefit from free hospital accommodation and the incredible camaradarie this brought. My medical career has always reinforced the idea that "if you want something doing, ask a busy person" as Medics at university and since have always amazed me with their ability to have many other projects, hobbies and social events to balance their busy jobs.

'I can't think of a job I haven't enjoyed (though there are no shortage of less-than-enjoyable shifts) and I've been fortunate to use my medical training to work abroad in Africa and New Zealand, to travel as an expedition doctor, and to work in the medical centre at Glastonbury. While the politics and unclear future of the NHS make me try to ensure that prospective medical students understand the uncertainty, I usually undo this good work by telling them of my travels, and making them immediately press "send" on their University application forms.

'Over recent years, changes in medical politics have impacted particularly on juniors. The previously-revered medical registrar has become the first point of contact for routine tasks and even non-medical "emergencies" like a bird flying in through a ward window.... This excessive demand understandably deters many from higher medical training. I've had countless conversations with juniors who are interested in medical specialty training but are put off by having to 'be the med reg'. This sadly results in ever-dwindling rotas, staff shortages and most importantly the loss of many amazing doctors from the medical specialties. At the same time, while working hour limits have improved safety and work-life balance, erosion of the traditional team has reduced continuity and the sense of belonging, while increasing bureaucracy has made training more of an administrative challenge. Political events such as the junior doctor contract dispute and strikes of 2016 have been hugely detrimental to junior morale, and an increasing sense of individual culpability is encouraging defensive practice rather than the balancing of risks and probabilities.

'This has escalated over recent years with a number of high-profile criminal prosecutions of doctors for gross negligence manslaughter in relation to medical error. An increasing public sense that human error is unacceptable (and indeed a belief that it is avoidable) in healthcare risks setting the patient safety agenda back by decades, as clinicians will be fearful of confessing to mistakes and near-misses. This is in direct contrast to both the NHS's professed blame-free culture, and to the duty of candour imposed since the Francis Report. It ignores the human factors which are so crucial to safe healthcare; a genuine culture of honest error reporting as in the aviation industry would revolutionise safety records. Until the NHS truly embraces this safety agenda and moves away from blame in relation to error, such mistakes will continue and are likely to increase. The greatest challenge the NHS currently faces is that of COVID-19. Hospital and critical care facilities have been escalated beyond what was previously imaginable, and both clinical and non-clinical staff have adapted willingly to enormous changes in work practices and pressures. As a respiratory physician I face the difficult challenge of caring for COVID-19 patients while also maintaining services for patients with lung cancer (my subspecialty area) and other non-COVID respiratory illness. Breaking bad news over the telephone rather than in person has become a sad 'new normal' in order to keep patients as safe as possible. We are seeing a concerning reduction in referrals for suspected lung cancer and I fully expect this to translate into poor outcomes in the coming months and years.

'Irrespective of this, I feel incredibly fortunate to work in such an interesting, varied and challenging profession, with some of the most dedicated people I can imagine. The NHS is, for all its faults, a fantastic institution of which the country is rightly proud. I believe passionately in the principle of healthcare free at the point of need and share Aneuryn Bevan's view that 'no society can legitimately call itself civilised if a sick person is denied medical aid because of lack of means'. This must be protected at all costs, whatever commercial and trade pressures may come in the post-Brexit world.

2019   **The NHS Long Term Plan** is published which sets out priorities for how the £20.5bn additional NHS funding promised by 2023/24 will be spent. The focus is on preventative medicine and making use of technology, with improvements promised in mental health, maternity and cancer care.

The Five year GP contract framework is agreed in line with the long term plan, with a focus on increasing the workforce, improving access and joining up care. A state backed indemnity scheme is introduced along with a £4.5bn annual investment in community services. CCGs are told to establish primary care networks to deliver these ideals.

NHSx is estalished by Matt Hancock to develop best practice for NHS technology. It brings together information technology teams from DHSC, NHSE and NHS Improvement to "make things better for patients and staff". The X stands for "user experience". Priorities are making it easier for patients to access NHS services on a smartphone and cutting time clinicians spend inputting and accessing data in NHS systems. The organisation manages the sharing of NHS data with industry. In 2020 NHSx commissioned a COVID-19 contct tracing app.

The interim NHS People Plan is publised in response to the gaping workforce gaps across the NHS. It calls for improvements in NHS culture and workforce planning

Theresa May resigns as Prime Minister and is replaced by Boris Johnson

2020   **The UK officially leaves the European Union**

COVID-19 is declared to be the greatest challenge the NHS has ever faced by Sir Simon Stevens NHS Englands CEO. Britain closes down as people are confined to their homes in lockdown. 'Nightingale' hospitals are rapidly constructed with the help of the armed forces, and retired clinicians and students are drafted in to assist with the pandemic response. GPs switch rapidly to remote consultations and routine dentistry is stopped. NHS England and NHS Improvement declare a Level 4 National Incident which allows them to order trusts to cancel elective care and discharge all patients who are medically fit to leave hospital.

Black Lives Matter protests held across the USA and three continents in response to the police killing unarmed black man George Floyd. In the UK, Bristol city centre statue of politician and slave trader Edward Colston is pulled down and pushed into Bristol Harbour.

Chapter 4

The Modern NHS

'I was to learn later in life that we tend to meet any new situation by re-organising, a wonderful method of creating the illusion of progress while producing inefficiency and demoralization'

Gaius Petronius – Roman Satirist 27-66AD

The NHS is a monolithic organisation, employing roughly 1.5 million people across the UK. The structure and administration of something so big is overwhelming. The sheer number of different organisations involved in the day to day running of the service is confusing even for those working within the service, especially given that these organisations have been renamed and rebranded each time a new government steps in, desperate to put their stamp on it. Seventy plus years of regular reforms with each successive government can be summed up in the quotation above.

For patients accessing the service, simply knowing where to go to seek help can be confusing. You stub your little toe and are worried it is broken – you go to your GP but can't get an appointment, the receptionist tells you that you will probably need an x-ray, which you can't get at the GP surgery. You go to hospital and wait four hours to be seen in A&E, only to be told by a grumpy triage nurse, that this isn't an emergency, you should have gone to the Minor Injuries Unit. You go to the minor injuries unit, and are told, you can have an x-ray, but there is a bit of a wait, and after looking at the toe, the treatment will be the same with or without an x-ray. Your toe gets strapped, and you think that you could have done that yourself by visiting the pharmacy for some tape.

To improve a health service in crisis, it is essential for everyone using it to have an understanding of how it works, to be empowered to make it better.

NHS UK

The NHS was UK-wide when it was established in 1948, but decentralisation in the late 1990s put control of all four nations health systems into the hands of each nation (England, Northern Ireland, Scotland and Wales), resulting in health service policies which are quite different. All of the UK has a tax funded service offering universal coverage, and the same core values. However, since devolution, reorganisations have occurred at different times, and policies have diverged. Prime examples of this can be seen by comparing England with Scotland. For example, free prescription drugs are provided, in Scotland, there is free personal social care for the over-65s and the purchase of NHS funded care from private hospitals is discouraged.

The NHS in England is the largest and most market-oriented of the four, and what follows, focuses on the structure of the English system.

NHS England

Since the NHS is funded by taxes, it is inextricably linked to the Government, and therefore politics. The Secretary of State for Health is head of the Department of Health – rebranded as the Department of Health and Social Care (DHSC) from January 2018. The Government creates national policies and legislation and decides how much money the NHS receives. The DHSC is supported by fifteen arm's length bodies (table 4.1) and a number of other agencies, external regulators and public bodies, which will be introduced below. Arm's length bodies are organisations that operate slightly apart from central government to conduct some of their business – meaning they are also easy to close down or re-organise if there are problems. They are also known as QANGOs (Quasi-Autonomous Non-Governmental bodies).

The bulk of the NHS piggybank goes to NHS England – an organisation that was created in 2013 as a result of the Health and

The NHS: The Story so Far

Table 4.1: The Department of Health and Social Care – Arm's length Bodies

NHS England	Leads the NHS in England by overseeing commissioning – the planning and buying of NHS services	https://www.england.nhs.uk
NHS Improvement	NHS Improvement oversees NHS trusts and independent providers to ensure high quality care which is, most importantly, financially sustainable. In April 2016, NHS Improvement was the rebranded name for the merging of 5 other organisations: -Monitor The regulator of NHS foundation trusts, which ensures they are financially sound and well governed -NHS Trust Development Authority (TDS) Formed in 2013 to be responsible for trusts unable to achieve foundation status -Patient Safety (including the National reporting and learning system (NRLS)) The National Patient Safety Agency (NPSA) was set up in 2001 to monitor patient safety incidents in a national database called the National Reporting and Learning System (NRLS). The NRLS allows similar incidents to be analysed to find common causes in an attempt to find solutions and avoid future incidents. NHS England took on the function of the NPSA in 2012, and NHS Improvement in 2016.	https://improvement.nhs.uk Monitor https://www.gov.uk/government/organisations/monitor NHS Trust Development Authority http://webarchive.nationalarchives.gov.uk/20161104155037/http://www.ntda.nhs.uk/ Patient Safety http://webarchive.nationalarchives.gov.uk/20160604124907/https://www.england.nhs.uk/patientsafety/ National reporting and learning system https://report.nrls.nhs.uk/nrlsreporting/Default.aspx

NHS Improvement	-Advancing Change Team Represented practical developmental learning programmes to help NHS staff and partner organisations to deliver change and improve services -Intensive Support Team Were external teams brought in to improve and support failing NHS organisations	Advancing change team http://webarchive.nationalarchives.gov.uk/20160506181459tf_/http://www.nhsiq.nhs.uk/capacity-capability/advancing-change.aspx Intensive support teams http://www.nhsimas.nhs.uk/ist/
Care Quality Commission	The CQC was previously known as the Healthcare Commission, and before that the Commission for Health Improvement and is essentially a regulatory body. The CQC monitors, inspects and regulates the standards of care provided by the NHS, local authorities, private companies and voluntary organisations, including independent hospitals, GP and dental surgeries, ambulance services and care homes.	http://www.cqc.org.uk
National Institute for Health and Care Excellence	Provides national guidance and advice to improve health and social care	https://www.nice.org.uk
Public Health England	Acts as the central organisation to lead public health initiatives such as health promotion, and immunization and screening programmes. Local health authorities took back responsibility for public health in 2013, and Public Health England provides overall leadership.	https://www.gov.uk/government/organisations/public-health-england
NHS Digital (previously known as Health and Social Care Information Centre)	The technological infrastructure of the NHS, uses data and technology to improve the NHS	http://content.digital.nhs.uk

(*Continues*)

Table 4.1 (*Continued*)

Health Education England	Delivers education and training for the entire NHS workforce. Made up of 6 advisory groups (to represent the interests of medical, dental, nursing, pharmacy, healthcare science and allied healthcare professionals) and 13 Local Education and Training Boards (LETB), who determine the local arrangements for the commissioning of education and training	https://www.hee.nhs.uk
Health Research Authority	Oversees health and social care research	https://www.hra.nhs.uk
NHS Blood and Transplant	Manages Blood donation and transplantation, researches new treatments and processes	http://www.nhsbt.nhs.uk
Medicines and Healthcare Products Regulatory Agency	Regulates medicines, medical devices and blood components in the UK	https://www.gov.uk/government/ organisations/medicines-and-healthcare-products-regulatory-agency
NHS Business Services Authority	Provision of central NHS services such as pensions schemes, payment of dentists and pharmacists, counter fraud, and determining the prices the NHS pays for consumables, including medication.	https://www.nhsbsa.nhs.uk NHS Pensions https://www.nhsbsa.nhs.uk/ nhs-pensions NHS help with costs https://www.nhsbsa. nhs.uk/nhs-help-health-costs NHS Prescription services https://www. nhsbsa.nhs.uk/nhs-prescription-services Information services https://www.nhsbsa.nhs. uk/information-services NHS penalty charges https://www.nhsbsa. nhs.uk/nhs-penalty-charges

NHS Business Services Authority		Student services https://www.nhsbsa.nhs.uk/student-services NHS Dental services https://www.nhsbsa.nhs.uk/nhs-dental-services Total rewards statements https://www.nhsbsa.nhs.uk/total-reward-statements NHS Injury Benefits Scheme https://www.nhsbsa.nhs.uk/nhs-injury-benefits-scheme Supplier Management https://www.nhsbsa.nhs.uk/supplier-management Infected blood support scheme https://www.nhsbsa.nhs.uk/england-infected-blood-support-scheme NHS Protect https://www.nhsbsa.nhs.uk/nhs-protect-1
NHS Resolution (previously known as NHS Litigation Authority)	Manages claims against the NHS, resolves concerns about NHS professionals (including both clinical negligence claims and general claims such a occupational injuries). This is funded by annual premiums from trusts. The National Clinical Assessment Service (NCAS) is an operating division of NHS resolution, which helps to resolve concerns about the professional practice of doctors, dentists and pharmacists.	http://www.nhsla.com/Pages/Home.aspx
Human Fertilisation and Embryology Authority	Independent regulator of fertility treatment and research	https://www.hfea.gov.uk
Human Tissue Authority	Regulation of organizations involved with human tissue removal, storage, education and research	https://www.hfea.gov.uk
NHS Counter Fraud Authority	Investigation and prevention of fraud and economic crime within the NHS	https://cfa.nhs.uk

Social Care Act of 2012, in an attempt to distance the NHS from politics. NHS England effectively leads the NHS in England, setting the priorities and direction of the service. It was created as an independent special health authority to distance politicians from any operational responsibility. NHS England oversees the commissioning, planning and buying of NHS services, sharing out over £100 billion in funds to the clinical commissioning groups (or CCGs) across the country. Some services, such as public health services, are commissioned directly by NHS England, but the bulk of commissioning is done by the CCGs.

NHS Commissioning

The planning of health services to meet the needs of the population has been necessary throughout th history of the NHS, but how this has been done has changed over time. Since the 1990s when the internal market was introduced, local commissioners became independent bodies with the powers and budgets to engage separate service providers to meet the needs of their own populations. Frequent reorganisation has taken place since then (see box 4.1) and the services have evolved to essentially do the same job, but have shuffled around those responsible for the delivery.

Box 4.1 The History of NHS Commissioning

Health Authorities and GP fundholding (1991-1999)
The introduction of the purchaser-provider split passed the responsibility for commissioning most health services to district health authorities. Groups of GP practices were given the option to control budgets to commission some services (such as elective hospital care and community services) but the health authorities retained overall responsibility

Locality Commissioning (1994-1999)
Alternative models to GP fundholding evolved in the nineties including locality commissioning, which relied on GPs and patients giving their input to the commissioning decisions via structured engagement, rather than GPs taking responsibility for delegated budgets.

Total Purchasing Pilots (1995-1999)
This offered groups of GP practices opportunities to commission more services-in theory, all hospital and community services. In practice, those participating focused on few key areas such as mental health and community services.

GP Commissioning (1998-1999)
The new Labour government replaced GP fundholding with GP commissioning which incorporated a range of different models, all which allowed GP practices to give their unput to the health authority commissioning decisions.

Primary Care Groups (1999-2002)
Prior to 1999, GP participation in commissioning was voluntary. Primary care groups were nationally mandated, and slowly took over commissioning from the district health authorities, with the aim that they would eventually become freestanding 'Primary Care Trusts'

Primary Care Trusts (2002-2013)
The NHS Plan 2000 envisioned PCGs becoming PCTs to take on the commissioning functions previously done by the health authorities. PCTs commissioned the bulk of health services, and also had powers to provide some community services themselves (such as district nursing, health visiting and children's services). They were also responsible for public health improvement.

Practice-based commissioning (2005-2013)
Designed to give primary care professionals the power to decide how NHS money is spent in their local area, GP practices were given virtual budgets to commission services, with the actual money still being controlled by the PCTs.

Clinical Commissioning Groups (2013-present)
Over 200 CCGs were created as a result of the 2012 Health and Social Care Act, replacing PCTs as the key local commissioning organisations. GPs were required to be members of their local CCG, and governing bodies had to be chaired by a clinician.

(adapted from http://www.kingsfund.org.uk/sites/default/files/2020-02/TBAC%20report%20%28web%29.pdf)

The current system for commissioning was implemented as a result of the Coalition government's Health and Social Care Act in 2012. The reforms created new organisations for the purchaser side, the provider side, and those to improve accountability for both (see table 4.2)

NHS England directly commissions specialised services, including renal dialysis, neonatal services and treatments for rare cancers. Primary care (including GPs, pharmacists, prison care, armed forces and dentists) and Public Health services are also directly commissioned. In 2016/17, NHS England had a commissioning budget of £105.9 billion. £28.2 billion was allocated for direct commissions, but the majority of this budget, £76.6 billion, wass allocated to local CCGs (see Fig 4.2).

Clinical Commissioning Groups, or CCGs, replaced Primary Care Trusts (PCTs) in April 2013, on the premise of moving the decision-making away from managers and back to clinicians. They have a statutory responsibility for commissioning most NHS services, such as emergency and urgent care, acute care, mental health and community services. They are increasingly involved in co-commissioning with NHS England some of the specialised services. Since 2015, NHS England has devolved responsibility for primary care to the CCGs – creating a

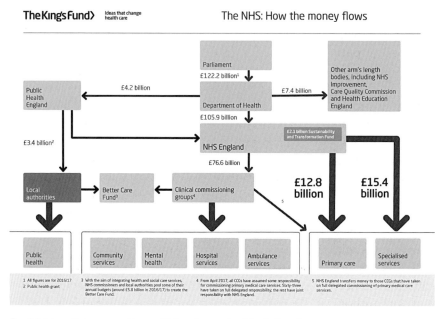

Fig 4.2 How the money flows. (Taken from the King's Fund)

Table 4.2: Summary of the Health and Social Care Act 2012

Purchaser Side	Clinical Commissioning Groups The National Commissioning Board (Renamed NHS England in April 2013)
Provider Side	Any Qualified Provider (AQP) Foundation Trusts
Regulators and Accountability	The Care Quality Commission (CQC) and Healthwatch England Monitor and Trust Development Agency (TDA) Health and Wellbeing Boards (HWB)

structural conflict of interests, whereby the supposedly GP run CCGs commission (i.e. pay) themselves.

When first established in 2013, there were 211 CCGs, responsible for an average of a quarter of a million people each (although some CCG populations range from 100,000 to 900,000). CCGs are made up of groups of local GP practices, which are led by an elected governing body (made up of GPs, nurses, secondary care clinicians and lay members). All GP practices have to be members of CCGs. This was a key principle of the 2013 reforms, which ministers used to defend the changes – as GPs were identified as the clinical group most aware of locals needs, priorities and services available, and most able to act as advocates for local communities. This sounds good in theory, but the reality of this is that overstretched GPs with a caseload of patients to care for, have little time or inclination to also take on the extra job of managing a budget of millions and planning services for their local areas. Most GPs opposed this, recognising they would be required to take the blame for rationing care to their own patients. In practice, CCGs are run by executive boards of managers, and GP involvement has been limited to small groups, rather than the GP community as a whole. Limited studies of CCGs have shown that the initial enthusiasm of some GP leaders to be involved had waned. A Lewisham GP wrote in the *Guardian* of the hours she spent acquiring the skills needed to lead commissioning in the local area, only to discover that the decision-making remained where it always had done – with the central managers. She felt the involvement of GPs was no more than window dressing for central planning geared towards the needs of the Foundation Trusts and private sector.

Local authorities are responsible for commissioning publicly funded social care services such as residential care and 'home help' services.

About £15 billion was spent on adult social care in 2016/17. Until the late 1980's, long term care of the elderly was financed through the NHS and social security entitlements. This was removed by Margaret Thatcher's government and became the responsibility of local council social service departments, and people became subject to means tested charges. Today, most people in care homes pay for most of the costs of their own care. In 1979, 64 per cent per cent of residential and nursing home beds were provided by the NHS or local authorities. By 2012, it was 2012, only 6 per cent per cent. Domiciliary services such as home help schemes have also been privatised. In 1993, 95 per cent of these services were provided directly by local authorities, and by 2012, it was just 11 per cent.

Local authorities are also responsible for the commissioning of the public health services not covered by NHS England, including sexual health services, health visitors, school nursing and addiction services. The public health grant for local authorities has been ring fenced (meaning it cannot be used for other purposes) and for 2019/20 was £3.1bn (in 2017/18 it was £3.3bn; in 2016/17 it was £3.6bn).

Health and Wellbeing Boards are formal committees that bring together local authorities and NHS representatives to carry out joint needs assessments with CCGs to develop joint strategies for their local populations.

CCGs and NHS England are supported by commissioning support units (CSUs) and from a range of private management consultants and voluntary sector organisations such as Capita, Optum and eMBED. These non-clinical support services are businesses which are themselves paid for by NHS money, to provide supporting back office services to the CCGs, such as IT, data management and HR support.

Any Qualified Provider (AQP)

To create a competitive market (especially for elective services), commissioners can procure from 'any qualified provider', which has opened the door for non-NHS private companies to profit from the system. This was introduced as early as 2004, following the GP contract changes, which led to private providers taking over GP out of hours care. All providers must be accredited and licensed by the CQC, but any organisation with the required competencies can compete for NHS-funded work. This was one of the most contentious issues of the 2012 reforms, meaning that the internal market (where NHS providers

How providers are regulated and commissioned. (Taken from the King's fund)

competed for business from NHS Primary Care Trusts) was no more. Instead, any organisation – private companies included – can compete for work. Common AQP services provided by private companies and third sector organisation (such as charities) include direct access MRI scanning, hearing aids and smoking cessation services. Private providers are notorious for cherry-picking less complex, more profitable patients and services, meaning that the NHS is left to deal with the more complex, costly cases that the private sector does not wish to provide (as it does not make money).

Sustainability and Transformation Plans (STPs)

From 2015, some more acronyms were thrown into the mix. Sustainability and Transformation Partnerships or Plans (STPs) describe geographic areas of CCGs, local authorities and other local health care services that have united to plan and deliver healthcare. Their aim is to re-organise healthcare in a way that suits the local population. Money saving is a key driver of the plans, and service cuts are expected in favour of more integration of care. From 2017, Integrated Care Systems (ICSs) or Accountable Care Systems (ACSs) have evolved to basically do the same thing, but with a new name. The Plain English Campaign criticised the language of these plans saying they are 'vague enough to hide all manner of changes', while the BMA has questioned if NHS leaders actually have the budgets available to deliver the proposed projects.

Primary Care Networks (PCNs)

The 2019 NHS Long-term plan aims for ICSs to cover the entire country by April 2021. This plan also introduced primary care networks which allow GP practices to come together to work at scale, which can aid with recruitment and staff retention, managing financial pressures and provide a range of services to patients. The Long-term plan has a vision that PCNs will deliver services that would not be feasible in smaller practices - such as first contact physiotherapy, extended access and social prescribing. Funding is planned to recruit physician associates, community paramedics and physiotherapists to extend the range of services available to patients and improve access.

NHS Finances

The money spent by the NHS is public money, raised from taxation. Each year, the government debates the annual budget, culminating in a vote to allocate money to the Department Health and Social Care, to spend on the health of the nation. The budget England in 2019/20 was an estimated £121 billion. This is out of an estimated £140.4 billion for the NHS in the UK as a whole.

Since 1948, spending on the NHS has risen on average by 3.7 per cent each year. In 1950, the NHS spent an estimated £460 million. In 2020, it will to spend over 300 times as much and the population has not risen 300-fold. Over this time period, increased costs and inflation would account for a lot of the spending, as well as increased medical innovations and more access to expensive technology and treatment. The ageing population has also contributed, as well as inefficiencies in how it is spent. To mark the 70th birthday of the NHS in 2018, the Prime Minister announced that funding for the NHS in England would be increased by £20.5bn by 2023/24 - or by an average of 3.4% per year (which was welcomed but increases of at least 4% a year are needed to meet the basic needs of the NHS).

How much a country spends on healthcare, is ultimately a political and societal choice. Ken Loach says in the book *NHS SOS*, 'if the political will to sustain a publicly funded health service existed, a way would be found. If it were simply a matter of finance, there are solutions to hand' – such as gathering the billions of pounds of unpaid and uncollected taxes, along with the trillions that exist off shore to be used for the common good.

But equally, we have a responsibility as users of the service, to remember it is not a bottomless pit. In the UK, we are pretty ignorant about what healthcare costs. As an NHS GP, I have been asked to prescribe (often for wealthy patients, eligible for free prescriptions because of their age) toothpaste, sunscreen, vitamins and an entire grocery list of gluten free products. We as patients get grumpy if the GP asks us to go and pay for a 19p packet of paracetamol from a supermarket or pharmacy instead of getting it on prescription. Perhaps an awareness of the bigger picture would help. In 2016, the NHS spent more than £70 million giving paracetamol out on prescription. Once dispensing, consulting and administration fees are factored in, a prescription for 32 paracetamol can cost the NHS £34. NHS England launched a consultation at the end of 2017 to try to curb this spending, by asking that routine prescribing for self-limiting conditions stops. An estimated £136million could be saved by doing this, which could be re-invested in other areas of the NHS. Annually, the NHS spend £4.5 million on shampoos for dandruff (enough to fund 4,700 cataracts operations or 1,200 hip replacement operations) £7.5 million on indigestion and heartburn (enough to fund 300 community nurses) and £5.5 million on mouth ulcers (1,500 hip replacements). Is this a slippery slope in itself, that will lead to the poorest being denied the prescriptions they need? there needs to be a balance. In 1948, I very much doubt that patients were picking up their gluten free pizza bases and biscuits for free during a visit to see their GP – times have changed, and the system does need to adapt to change as well. Does paying your taxes really entitle you to free toothpaste on prescription for your holiday to Myanmar (for which you have got first class seats)? – true story.

Perhaps this money could be spent instead on the woefully underfunded mental health services. More than 4,000 mental health beds have closed since 2010, coupled with a similar reduction in the number of psychiatric nurses. Access to these services is dire, as one service user recalls of her experience as an inpatient:

> 'I do feel in 2018 that mental health issues are talked about
> a lot more, which is as it should be. Life on a ward is grim –
> you tend to walk around in circles trying to get cigarettes,

tears, people screaming. We were all so unwell and had been removed from society. I have been sectioned at various times over the past 40 years. Many locked wards that I've been on were tragically understaffed. It was an extremely unhealthy environment, with a shortage of compassion. If I became ill again today, I would find it very difficult to get a bed. I would need to travel more than 40 miles as so many psychiatric wards have been shut. On the upside, I have a decent enough mental health team, who I have a lot of faith in, but their job is difficult, with staff often off on long term sick.'

Regulation of Professionals

Individual professionals within the NHS are regulated through bodies such as the General Medical Council (GMC), the Nursing and Midwifery Council, the Health Professions Council, the General Dental Council, the General Optical Council and the General Osteopathic Council. The Royal Colleges and Specialist societies are membership organisations who have a range of responsibilities for ensuring standards of training in their particular areas, as well as improving service delivery.

The GMC

The GMC is the independent regulator of doctors in the UK. It is a registered charity whose purpose is to protect the public by ensuring good standards of medical education and practice. The GMC was formed under the Medical Act of 1858 in response to a census at the time, which suggested that a third of all doctors in England were unqualified. Today, it maintains a register of qualified doctors, including a specialist register of consultants and general practitioners – for which all doctors pay an 'annual retention fee' to maintain their name on the register. At the end of the seventies, this fee was £10 per annum from April 2020 it was £406, and failure to pay the fees can result in erasure from the register. The GMC sets standards for medical education for medical schools and ensures doctors stay up to date through Continuing Professional Development, and since 2012, through revalidation (see chapter 3). The Medical Act gives the GMC powers to take measures if questions are raised about a doctor's fitness to practise. Revalidation was introduced as a more proactive way of requiring doctors to demonstrate they are fit to practise and takes place every five years. Doctors who fail to engage with this will find themselves unable to practice. However the infrastructure of revalidation is almost entirely provided by the NHS – meaning that doctors without regular NHS employment, who may have previously plugged rota gaps, or provided NHS services in other ways, are unable to do so as easily as before. During the COVID-19 pandemic, revalidation was put on hold, giving doctors a breather from the process, to concentrate their time on dealing with the outbreak.

Since the Nineties, trust in the medical profession has declined following scandals such as Shipman, Bristol and Mid Staffs. However, the knee jerk reaction of stronger regulation to prevent this is not entirely evidence based, and the impact this has on professional motivation, and the health system as a whole is not insignificant. Doctors can be referred to the GMC by anyone, with no redress for groundless referral. Between 1992-2012, complaints to the GMC against doctor rose eight-fold. The number of public hearings increased five-fold, while the number of doctors erased from the medical register increased twelve-fold. Between 2003-2013, 96 doctors died while undergoing fitness to practice procedures (how many of these were suicide is unknown). In line with this inflation of claims, medical defence organisations (which all doctors are obliged to be members of) have increased their fees year on year to maintain cover for members subject to a GMC enquiry. The GMC itself acknowledges that there is no evidence of a decline in standards of medical practice to justify their increased activity. Furthermore, there is no published evidence, that GMC fitness to practise processes improve the quality of medical care given to patients. There is evidence however, that a complaint culture results in the practice of defensive medicine. Doctors dealing with claims often give up clinical practice, or report feeling more distant from their patients. Most tragically of all, many clinicians facing investigation have taken their own lives. The question must therefore be asked – is the GMC fit to practice, when its own activity seems to take no regard of its impact on both doctors and patients?

NHS Staff

The NHS is haemorrhaging staff. As the workload and conditions become worse, more and more undervalued staff opt to throw in the towel to go elsewhere. Figures from OECD show that the UK has fewer doctors per head than most of Europe – 2.8 doctors per 1000 people, which is below the OCED average of 3.4. Like the Eurovision results, we perform poorly compared to most of our neighbours such as Greece who has the most at 6.1, but Portugal (4.6), France (3.3), Estonia (3.4) and Latvia (3.2) all fare better than us. The NHS is desperately short of nurses, and figures from early 2018 show that across England, only 1 in 7 of all empty nursing posts were filled. GPs too, face a recruitment crisis, and despite a government pledge to increase GP numbers by 5000 by 2020, the number of full time equivalent GPs fell by 0.3 per cent per cent in 2016. GP workload has grown in recent years, not only in volume, but in complexity, and experienced GPs are seeking early retirement, whilst newly qualified GPs opt for portfolio careers, combining clinical work with teaching, research, or anything other than the daily slog of full time GP work. Given the long training times for clinical professionals, there are concerns over whether the NHS can recruit and retain enough staff to meet the growing demands on the service.

Those staff that remain are undervalued. Junior doctors in particular, are uniquely exploited by management, who are aware that they are unlikely to complain and risk their future employment at a trust. Junior doctors have often been doctors for many years, but until they become a consultant, training programmes mandate them to rotate to different hospitals every 3-12 months. This in itself can be isolating and demoralising, working shifts with different colleagues each day, with no time to build relationships before moving on again. Trainees are routinely posted to work in hospitals miles away from their homes – often only getting their rotas a few days prior to a changeover. Rota gaps are expected to be covered. Some surgical trainees are required to work a full day and then be on call overnight – sometimes from home. Some hospitals have mandated these doctors to remain on the hospital site overnight if their homes are too far away – and in these cases, on call rooms are provided by the hospital. One surgical registrar spoke of being sent a bill for the use of this room and threatened with debt collectors if he did not pay. Worried about his career, he paid, for a room he was too busy to use, a room that would be sitting empty anyway, and a room he didn't want in the first place.

My NHS Story

Dr Neil Barnard is a South African medical graduate who completed his intensive care and emergency medicine training within the NHS. He recently moved his family over to New Zealand to live and work, and he shares his reasons why.

'I came to work in the NHS initially via the UK private system, followed by a stint as a ship's physician in the Caribbean, followed by further experience in South Africa, and training in Australia after which, having met my English wife, begrudgingly returning to England to live and work there.

'I am not wedded to the NHS because of some sort of national pride, political ideology or religious fervour. I was, in fact, a reluctant NHS worker when I first arrived to take up an emergency medicine post in Coventry. I was under no illusions when I left Australia to go to the UK. I knew that my lifestyle would be much worse, my pay would be no better and the weather would be abysmal. Yet, despite this, I was excited to have the opportunity to work in a system which valued doctors, was

Midlands Junior Doctors outside the Department of Health (Neil Barnard second from right, back row) (Photo taken by Matt Saywell - copyright of the British Medical Association)

consistently rated as one of the most efficient in the world, put patients before profit and would provide excellent, world class training.

'I arrived in the August of 2010, incidentally, three months after the Conservative Party became the major part of a coalition government.

'My first professional experience of the NHS was very rewarding, I worked in a motivated, extremely busy Emergency Department which had been newly built in the last five years. The workload, though intense was neither demoralising nor unmanageable. I worked with a group of colleagues and senior clinicians who were supportive of each other and felt rewarded in the work they did. Most importantly, the nursing staff were mostly, staff who had been in the department for a number of years and formed a stable and caring base upon which the department was built.

'So, what happened between then and August 2017 when, in the space of just seven years, despite having lived in the UK, bought a house, and had children who were starting to settle in school, I discussed matters with my wife and took the big decision to relocate our family to New Zealand? New Zealand was a country where neither of us had ever been; where we had neither friends nor family and where it would take either of us a day and a half of flying to get home if necessary.

'In short, the NHS had begun a slow and apparently unchecked spiral towards an underfunded, under-resourced service. A decline which allowed pay for NHS workers to be frozen for seven years resulting in a real term cut for some staff of 30 per cent. A decline which allowed the NHS budget, despite claims to the contrary, to be cut in real terms, when demands for acute services had never been higher yet staff numbers in terms of staff per attendance ratio had never been lower.

'In an unprecedented event in 2016, junior doctors, a largely homogenous group of uncomplaining, professional people who happily stayed extra hours and sacrificed their own time and effort for the good of their patients, went on strike – not over pay but in protest against the way the NHS has been eroded. Staff have been unsupported and conditions have deteriorated to a point where patient safety has been compromised as a result of doctors not being able to provide the level of care they want to for their patients.

'In the last two years, we have heard countless news stories about nurses using food banks to survive to the end of the month and nurses being balloted about potential strike action. In my own department, nursing turnover was so high that having spent 18 months doing subspecialty training in a different department, I returned to find that I no longer knew most of the nurses working there. Burnout, exhaustion and record numbers of staff retirements and absence due to sickness have all lead to a massive reliance on locum staff who neither know or care for the departments they work in.

'By the time, I had come to the end of my training in the UK and despite having a dual qualification in intensive care and emergency medicine which afforded me the pick of jobs anywhere in the country, I could not face working feeling as if my back were constantly against the wall. I could not face feeling as if we were shuffling the deck chairs on the *Titanic* while our politicians instructed the band to play on, oblivious of the looming crisis.

'It turns out, I left at the right time. I am still a member of the local trainee group at my former hospital trust. It is heart breaking this year to hear stories of patients piled up in corridors, of record ambulance waits, of record waiting times to be seen in the department and hearing the stories of mental, physical and emotional exhaustion in my colleagues who are some of the hardest working people I've had the privilege to work with. It galls me more when on the BBC news, the politicians of the day, can only talk about how well they were prepared for the winter. It is clear that they were never prepared and their empty thanks for the hard work being put in by NHS workers across the spectrum of care feel like empty platitudes.

'Perhaps I should not have been surprised when I arrived in New Zealand and found that 60 per cent per cent of the junior medical staff in my new department were UK graduates. I should also not have been surprised that almost all of them have no plans to return to the country of their birth. When one considers the differences in conditions, it really isn't surprising at all.

'We work in a department where staff numbers are adequate and necessary resources are provided. Nursing numbers follow recommendations applied by the Australasian College of Emergency Medicine. Training is an integral part of the system and consultant staff have the time to teach while junior staff have the time to be taught.

'A work/life balance is recognised as a vital part of staff happiness and productivity such that sickness rates are much lower and staff are motivated and keen to come to work. The hospital trust recognises the work that we do and values us sufficiently to pay for professional indemnity, professional registration and ongoing clinical development.

'The work is certainly not of a lesser standard or complexity. I am challenged daily but, importantly, I feel supported by my colleagues, the hospital and the Health Service as a whole. It appears that the system that was largely based on NHS principles and has always looked up to the NHS has now got much to teach the NHS in return.

'I have no desire to return to the NHS unless a fundamental commitment is made which will help turn things around. Until then, I can look forward to the ongoing steady stream of former colleagues sending me their CVs and asking about vacancies.

'Shame. The once proudest achievement of post war Britain is no more. How the mighty have been allowed to fall.'

Please Let Us Work

Amidst our NHS workforce crisis, where GP leaders and politicians proclaim that urgent measures should be taken to invest in recruitment to boost GP numbers, there exists a cohort of qualified GPs who are desperate to return to the UK to work as GPs but are being strangled by red tape.

Any doctor wishing to work as an independent, unsupervised GP in the UK, is required to:

1 be on the GMC GP Register (which means completing 5-6 years of medical school, and working at least 5 years as a doctor)
2 Hold a GMC licence to practise
3 Be on the National Performers' list

There are three performers' lists operated by NHS England (for medical, dental and ophthalmic performers) that exist to provide another layer of reassurance for the public that professionals practising in the NHS are suitably qualified, with up to date training, can speak English and have passed relevant checks (such as with the Disclosure and Barring Service [DBS]). Performers' lists came into operation in April 2004 (a result of the Health and Social Care Act [Community Health and Standards] 2003), as a reaction to cases of dodgy doctors in the NHS (notably, Shipman), to create a formal process to ensure quality.

This means that experienced GPs who did not train in the UK, and doctors who have been out of UK general practice for two years, must jump through a series of expensive and time consuming hoops before they can join or re-join the NHS workforce. Overseas doctors must first obtain the Certificate of Eligibility for GP Registration (CEGPR) – a process that often takes up to twelve months, collecting documents and providing evidence. Instead of reviewing each doctor on a case by case basis, and considering their experience and merits, both overseas doctors and returning UK doctors then all have to go through the GP Induction and Refresher Scheme (I&R Scheme) – another process which can take a further twelve months to navigate. Having these safeguards is understandable, to ensure GPs working in the UK are familiar with the NHS and are up to date after long periods out of practice. But blindly subjecting all returning GPs to the same process if they do have the experience and qualifications is a waste of valuable time and resources which could be better spent providing a service to the public and reducing GP waiting times. To add insult to injury, this process costs money. To obtain the CEGPR, one doctor calculated expenses of over £2,000 for the whole process, and for the I&R scheme, almost £5,000 – not including the loss of income for the entire time they were not working. Many GPs opt to remain overseas, or throw in the towel completely, and pursue alternate careers, rather than put themselves through this process. Is it any wonder we have no GPs, if coming back to work in the UK is so much hassle?

GP I&R Scheme Case Study

Dr Irina Bardsley qualified as a UK GP in 2013, after completing a formal three year speciality training programme in the North of England as a GP Registrar. She co-authored a book to help fellow trainees pass one of the exams required to become a GP, and then went to work as a GP in New Zealand for three years with her husband.

During her three year period away from UK general practice, she worked continuously as a general practitioner in New Zealand in what the GMC and Medical Council of New Zealand (MCNZ-NZ's GMC equivalent) describe as a 'comparable healthcare system'. She was required – as part of the MCNZ's registration requirements – to be enrolled in a portfolio system almost identical to those used in the UK to revalidate and appraise doctors. This involved completing a minimum set of annual CPD activities, audits, multi-source feedback, and patient feedback cycles. She maintained her registration with the GMC, but, on the advice of her UK appraisal lead, resigned from the performers list.

She returned to the UK for family reasons in 2017, with two job offers before she had even booked her flights home. She returned to the city in which she had trained, where practices had struggled to recruit

139

GPs for years. She was known to the staff and patients she would be working for. Her local performers' list invited her to a meeting to review her documents and welcomed her with open arms, thrilled that a UK-trained GP had returned to the country. The day before she was due to start working at the surgery, the performers list contacted her again to say sorry ... but she had been out of the UK for too long and could not work until she had completed the I&R scheme. The performers' list staff actually had no idea what was required and were unable to provide any guidance. This was the beginning of a lengthy process of paperwork, assessments, and mindless red tape which meant she was unable to work as a GP for more than six months.

The I&R scheme decided that anyone who had not served a minimum of two years working as a GP *prior* to moving overseas, does not qualify for the 'Portfolio Route' whereby Irina's evidence could have been reviewed to allow her to continue working in the same country that she trained and qualified in. Instead of looking at each individual doctor's circumstances, on a case-by-case basis, to allow those that have an exceptional level of evidence to simply continue to practice medicine, the scheme stops good doctors from working.

For Irina, what came next, was a series of demoralizing assessments, a simulated surgery exam – similar to the exam she had written a book about – and then supervised placements. Firstly there were clinical multiple choice questions, aimed at more junior doctors working in a hospital setting 'imagine you are an SHO in A&E or an F2 on the ward...' and questions about procedures that would never be carried out in primary care such as (consenting patients for specialist surgical procedures, or thrombolysing a pulmonary embolism). For an exam that is supposed to be geared up for GPs that are fully qualified and practicing, it is questionable this is fit for purpose. Following this was a Situational Judgment test, where candidates are asked to rank their actions in order of appropriateness. Actual questions include: 'a patient's dog has passed away, would you: advise her to get a dog from the shelter; give her one of your puppies that your own dog recently had; ask her to seek support from a friend?...' or 'A nurse asks you to help move furniture from one room to another while you are doing your surgery, please rank in order...'

How is this a superior method of assessing a GP's competence than reviewing actual evidence supplied from a medical council from another country with a similar healthcare system? The scheme is arguably a detriment to a doctor's clinical practice, in that they are removed from day to day clinical contact with patients for several months, to spend time relearning questions to pass an exam.

Working abroad arguably makes people better GPs, not worse. In some countries, it is actually encouraged to spend time working abroad before being fully signed off in a speciality. There is no other speciality in the UK that requires additional assessments to get back to work (including independently practicing medical consultants) – Irina's husband, for example was able to simply pick up where he left off three years earlier in hospital medicine, without the rigorous scrutiny and loss of earnings imposed on GP returners.

The I&R scheme is damaging the morale of previously enthusiastic GPs, keen to bring their overseas experiences back to the NHS, but find they are unable to work due to numerous (and arguably unnecessary) assessments. Even GP registrars in training are allowed to work independently (under the supervision of an allocated GP). So why is it so difficult for fully qualified GPs to return to practice, particularly those who haven't even had any time out? Why can't the scheme allow GP returners to arrange their own jobs (effectively being screened by an individual GP practice) and simply complete a minimum period of supervision without unnecessary exams? These are forcing them to take time out of practice, placing undue and unfair strain on good GPs from a financial, practical, and even mental-health perspective?

Private Healthcare and the USA

The Commonwealth Fund reported in 2014 that the NHS was rated top on quality of care and access to care, while the US, where the private sector provides healthcare, was the most expensive and the worst performing. The US assigns 18 per cent of its economy to health spending – double that of the UK, but is near the bottom in terms of health and life expectancy compared with sixteen other economically wealthy countries.

Healthcare costs in the USA are notoriously steep. In many hospitals, doctors' pay depends upon the procedures their patients have – meaning that financial incentives can impact on the care given. As George Bernard Shaw wrote at the turn of the twentieth century, giving people a financial interest in cutting your leg off can have some pretty obvious drawbacks. A colleague in the States spoke of a medical bill amounting to $86,000 when his father passed away at home, and healthcare professionals did little more than declare him dead. His family called 911 when his father collapsed with a cardiac arrest. The paramedics charged a fee for every mile it took them to reach his home in the ambulance, in addition to the fee charged to dial 911 in the first place. They charged for the act of unloading their equipment from the ambulance, a fee to enter the house, another charge for starting CPR, for picking him up from the floor to a stretcher, more costs to move him to the ambulance, charges to open their bag and for every medication and disposable item used during their visit – even down to the gloves worn by the paramedics and the piece of paper used to cover the stretcher his father lay on. The fee to declare him dead alone was $7,000.

A day in hospital in the US costs over ten times more than in other countries and patients get more tests and more interventions – driven by profit and fear of litigation, rather than from practising good medicine. Instead of sharing risk and uncertainty, patients are over-investigated and over-treated. Popular doctors will attract more customers, and popular doctors will often be the ones that give customers what they want. Antibiotics for their runny nose that started this morning; IV opioid analgesia for the sprained ankle … I previously worked as a cruise ship doctor for an American company. On cruise ships, guests pay for the medical services they receive. They also fill out guest satisfaction surveys at the end of their vacation where they rate the cruise. The fact they ended up in the medical facility already means they probably didn't enjoy their vacation due to being unwell, and then when we don't provide a 'Z-pack' (antibiotics) or Vicodin (narcotic) on request, or even worse if we isolate them for public health reasons to prevent an outbreak – we will hear about it in the survey. Similar 'rate my doctor' surveys exist in the US, and it is easy to see how as a doctor, it is easier to give a patient what they want to keep them happy (boosting ratings and profits) rather than having a difficult conversation – but this is not good medicine. To take the example of antibiotic prescribing – most of the guests with a cold on the ship came to see me expecting to be able to pay for antibiotics (antibiotics are not needed for a self-limiting illness – Public Health England have developed antibiotic guardian resources if you want to read more http:// antibioticguardian.com/). It would have been much easier for me to smile and hand them over, than to take the time to explain the reasons why they were not needed or unlikely to make them feel better – it risks confrontation and the likelihood of being blamed on the satisfaction survey for coughing for the entire vacation. Similar dilemmas arise in the NHS, and GPs have been threatened with being reported to the GMC for refusing to prescribe antibiotics for a cold.

At the opposite end of the private medicine spectrum, were the situations on board, where we were compelled to discuss the cost of treatment with patients to ensure they were happy to pay the fees. The medication used to bust the clot causing a heart attack costs $7,000. I have been in a situation where the patient was in a critical condition and I was stopped by the nurse to go and check with the person paying the bill that they were happy for us to administer this potentially life-saving treatment, at a cost of $7,000. In the NHS we don't have to worry about these issues …yet.

A study in the NEJM in 1997, concluded that almost 100,000 people died in the United States each year because of a lack of medical care, due to being unable to pay for medical insurance. Insurers limit their risks by selecting out the poor, the elderly, those with mental health problems, homeless people and migrants. Even amongst those who are insured, many fall ill, only to find they have inadequate coverage, and have to live with the fear of healthcare bills.

NHS Privatisation

Private companies have been part of the NHS for decades. It started in the eighties with support services such as portering, catering, cleaning and IT being provided by private companies. Following the 2004 GP contract changes, which allowed non-NHS providers to provide primary care services, private companies such as Virgin started to take over GP out of hours services. (see box 4.2) The following year, Independent sector treatment centres were introduced. The scale of private companies' involvement in the NHS accelerated following the 2012 Health and Social Care Act, to involve GP surgeries, urgent care and minor injuries units, community services, maternity care, ambulances, diagnostic imaging, prison care and even whole hospitals and A&E departments. Private consultancy firms are increasingly being used in health planning – in the form of commissioning support units and accountable care organisations. In 2016/17, almost 70 per cent of the 386 clinical contracts put out to tender went to the private sector (worth £3.1 billion), with Care UK and Virgin Care holding the largest share of these. This may not be obvious to patients using the service, since all these private providers are encouraged by the Department of Health's branding team to use the NHS logo, without using their own.

Box 4.2 GP Out-of-hours (OOH) Services

GPs are contracted to be responsible for their patients between 8am and 6.30pm Monday to Friday. OOH care is the service provided outside of these times.

Historically, GPs were responsible for their patients 24/7. They typically managed the out of hours period by forming co-operatives with other GPs to share the overnight and weekend calls.

Following the 2004 GP contract changes, which passed the responsibility for OOH GP services from the doctors to the primary care trusts, most GP practices opted out of this work. Many PCTs worked with the GP co-operatives (which eventually morphed into social enterprises). Some PCTs gave the OOH contracts to commercial providers such as Harmoni and Serco (who both were criticised for failing to employ enough doctors to run their service).

The National Audit Office carried out a survey of the urgent care system in England in 2014 and found that 26 per cent of the general public had never heard of GP OOH services and many more had no idea how to make contact.

NHS England issued guidance in 2015 to integrate NHS 111 and GP OOH services, meaning patients in need of care would have just one number to ring wherever they are in the country (111).

NHS 111 is staffed by trained health advisors (non-clinicians) who use the NHS Pathways triage tool to support patients. Approximately 70-80per cent of patients are triaged to have contact with a clinician outside of the 111 service. To reduce inefficiency and to provide a patient with a complete episode of care, from 2017, an integrated urgent care clinical assessment service (IUC CAS) was introduced, meaning a senior GP is available (who can electronically prescribe if needed) alongside advanced nurse practitioners, paramedics, pharmacists and dental nurses.

When COVID-19 hit in 2020, NHS 111 was commissioned to provide a dedicated COVID-19 Clinical Assessment Service (CCAS) to free up other areas of the healthcare system to manage those most at risk of complications. Many GPs came out of retirement to staff the service. According to NHS Digital, there were 2,962,751 calls to NHS 111 in England in March 2020 (compared to 1,503,318 in January).

Is this a problem? Yes. The priority of private companies is to provide a profit for the shareholders, meaning when it comes to healthcare, they are unlikely to get involved with services that are expensive to deliver. While the UK public sector continues to be cut back, the services deprived of the resources, such as emergency care, care for the elderly and the chronically sick, are the areas that private providers avoid at all costs, since they are complex, risky and unprofitable. Private hospitals in the UK, on the whole, are set up to treat elective cases – typically healthy patients undergoing routine, less risky procedures. UK private hospitals are not required to teach or train their staff. The headlines that undermine the NHS often put the alternative option of private care on a pedestal, as if poor care couldn't possibly happen there. I recall as a junior doctor, working in an NHS hospital, having private patients transferred to the care of the NHS as soon as they became too unwell to handle. Even as a GP, I was visiting a patient having chest pain in a rural area who asked me as we waited for the ambulance if they should use their insurance to go to a private hospital for treatment. My answer was no – the local private hospitals are fine for your routine knee replacement, but they are not where you want to be if you are acutely unwell with a likely heart attack. It is not possible to deliver universal healthcare through a market system, as it makes no money. To quote author Simon Sinek: "When people are financially invested, they want a return. When people are emotionally invested, they want to contribute". This is why a publicly funded and owned NHS is seen as amongst the fairest and most efficient in the world – when funded properly.

Medicine and the Media

The media shoulder a huge responsibility when it comes to informing the public about the NHS and about healthcare in general. How information is reported has an influence on people's perceptions – as was demonstrated during the MMR vaccine scare (where media coverage did not align with the weight of scientific evidence, leading to unvaccinated children and re-emergence of measles). As COVID-19 was declared a public health emergency in early 2020, the director-general of the World Health Organisation also declared that the world was suffering from an "infodemic" – an overabundance of information about the disease, some accurate and some not, making it harder to access reliable information.

Sadly, the vast majority of mainstream media reporting on the NHS is scaremongering propaganda, peddled by the politicians. At the start of the outbreak, NHS staff were hailed as heroes fighting the covid war. As Autumn approached, with cases back on the rise and a failed track and trace system causing chaos, the headlines reverted to GP bashing, diverting the blame away from government failings and onto primary care.

A study at Cardiff university in 2007 found that journalists were producing more content than they were 20 years before, but only 12 per cent of stories were being properly checked. Complexity, details and accuracy are compromised, and the speed at which erroneous or unfair allegations can be published has far reaching implications. Journalists work to deadlines, and it is easier to regurgitate a government press release, than to wade through the rhetoric to report the facts. Furthermore, explaining the complexity of the problems in the NHS, is going to take more than the 500 words allocated to most reporters. The NHS winter crisis, which has extended into a year-round problem, is a result of the government imposing years of austerity measures. Insufficient hospital beds and a lack of social care to discharge the patients in said beds, means the new patients attending A&E are stuck on trolleys for hours. The money that should have been spent on these services, was instead wasted on the NHS reorganisations designed to privatise the NHS. The Department of Health controls the health news agenda, and their press releases blame the inappropriate attendees, the GPs and the hospital managers and their solution is for the public to realise we need to start to pay for our care – scare tactics designed by the government to push forward their agenda of privatisation.

Journalists love human interest stories, and when it comes to the NHS there is an endless supply. Doctor bashing in particular, has become a national sport, reaching a peak during the recent junior doctor strikes. In a post-Shipman world, allegations against doctors make good copy, and are justified in the public interest. Poor care should rightly be flagged and rectified, but there are always several sides to a story. Patients who sell their stories are not bound by any codes of confidentiality. Whereas healthcare professionals certainly are bound by them, meaning correcting inaccuracies in the story may risk breaching confidentiality, and the true events of any scandal may not be what make the headlines.

The GMC has investigated doctors based on nothing more than a media report. An NHS colleague spent some time working for an online pharmacy, which was regulated by the CQC, with safeguards in place for prescribing over the internet. A journalist, in search of a story, placed a fraudulent request to the site, requesting the weight loss pill Orlistat. They filled out the online questionnaire which checks medical history, height, weight, contraindications to the medication and asks patients to confirm they are telling the truth. The journalist lied about their weight and height, saying they were obese when they had a normal BMI. The pill was provided, a scathing article was published, and the doctor prescribing the pill was referred to the GMC for further investigation. Where is the accountability for the actions of the journalist?

My NHS Story

Carol Trow is a full time author and editor who previously worked for the NHS and in the private sector until 2000 as a biomedical scientist. She shares her experiences as a user of the service, in a blog post that was originally written for the *Huffington Post* – 'No one wants to hear the NHS good news!'

'Five weeks ago, the unthinkable happened, right there, on the sofa; my previously healthy husband had a heart attack. I dialled 999 and dragged him off the sofa in one movement and within seconds was performing CPR. And screaming at him. Then the paramedics arrived and I heard the dreaded word – "Clear!" – and then silence; I have to admit, for a while there, it's a bit of a blur.

'Then suddenly, he was away from me, in an ambulance and the chaos that is A&E awaited. But … and here comes the bit that news media doesn't want to hear … the staff were all fabulous, the care he got was exemplary. There were no trollies in the corridors, no dirt, no mess, no waiting. Just a team all gathered round him, adding tubes and leads; arranging a bed in a nearby centre of excellence; sorting an Air Ambulance. Reception staff were patient, while dealing with dingbat members of the public abusing them because my husband had "jumped the queue".

I was hugged, consoled, told the truth – he might not make it, but if he didn't, it wasn't going to be because he wasn't fighting or that I had done anything wrong in the CPR. He was packed up like a Christmas parcel and loaded onto the helicopter on the way to Queen Alexandra Hospital, in Cosham.

'And then, the waiting. And the discovery that, pressured and beleaguered though it is, the NHS can really pull out all the stops, if you do the same. My husband, chilled to 36 degrees, intubated, sedated, with a balloon pump to keep his heart going, perhaps didn't look as if he was bringing much to the table, but my word, that man's a fighter. My son and his wife and baby son were with us on the long trip back to normal. And all the time, the nurses and doctors were by our side, caring, professional and I don't hesitate to say loving. We got attached to "our" first nurse, Ben, who quietly changed his next shift so he would be there next day as well. There was Liz, Edwin, Christian, Francisco, Claire, May, Edgar, Peter, David ... the list is endless of people who know their jobs inside out and how to go the extra mile.

'We were warned that we might not get "him" back, except in body as he may have had oxygen deprivation in the first minutes after the attack. But, he *is* back. He doesn't remember the actual event or the few days before it and his memory of his hospital stay is sketchy to absent, but everything else is fine; fine because someone in that A&E saw that he could make it; because the air ambulance and two centres of excellence were there; that the nurses, doctors, physios, all gave their time and love without condition. And because he wasn't ready to go – but spirit alone is nothing without the NHS.

'So – NHS knockers; Stop It! Time wasters – go to your pharmacy if you feel a bit under the weather. Read what it says on the sign; "Accident and Emergency". It doesn't say "Feeling a bit iffy and want some medicine". Cussers and swearers – keep it to yourself.

Being writers, we thought, hey – let's get to the media, tell them how fabulous everyone has been. We're not uber-famous, but eighty books is no small feat. He's been on telly as well, so we thought that the local media at least would print this feel-good story. But no. We didn't even get a phone call, an email in reply. It turns out that good news is no news.

'If we have learned anything, it is this. Don't listen to all the news about lines of grandmas left to languish on trollies in corridors. Don't listen to the stories about filth and "third world care". Listen to the *real* news that isn't news, that the NHS is alive and well – if a little underfunded. And get out there, do what you can to help the funding. We write, so that's what we're going to do. Our daughter-in-law is doing a run. Our son is putting on an all-day music fund raiser. Everyone can do something to help. But most of all, love and cherish our NHS – like the NHS, 70 years old this year and feeling her age, loves and cherishes us.

The Future

Is the NHS going to make it to its 80th birthday celebrations? Of course it will. The NHS is a set of principles about the way we value healthcare. It borders on being a national religion and still retains huge public support.

The report 'How good is the NHS' was compiled for the NHS's 70th birthday in 2018 and used OCED data and other sources to compare the NHS to healthcare systems in 18 similar countries. It's key strength is the financial protection it offers the public from the consequences of falling ill. Compared to other countries, the NHS also does well managing patients with some longterm conditions such as diabetes and kidney disease, with fewer hospital admissions reported.

As we all know without reading a report, there is room for much improvement. The NHS performed worse than average in the treatment of some of the most common causes of death. It has consistently higher rates of perinatal mortality, and is the third poorest performer (out of 18 developed countries) on rates of amenable mortality (which means potentially preventable premature deaths if timely and effective care is provided – eg. appendicitis).

To improve the NHS, we need to be better informed about what is going on. Many campaign groups have emerged since the Health and Social Care Act was passed (Keep Our NHS Public; the NHS Support Federation; 38 Degrees…) and they have an abundance of information on their websites – there is even a new political party, the National Health Action Party. To echo some of the suggestions posed by these groups, on how to 'Save the NHS', here are some practical things that we can all consider doing to ensure it reaches Eighty:

1. Join an NHS campaign group to engage in discussions about local issues (such as hospital closures/cuts). The NHS Support Federation provides details on how to campaign (nhscampaign.org) and the following NHS campaign groups are worth checking out:

A Better NHS https://abetternhs.net/about/
Centre for Health and the Public Interest – Independent health think tank http://chpi.org.uk
Keep our NHS public – Campaigns for the NHS https://keepournhspublic.com/ (accessed May 2018)

The NHS Support Federation – Pressure group that campaigns for the NHS http://www.nhscampaign.org

The National Health Action Party – Campaigns for the NHS https://nhaparty.org

Patients4NHS – www.patients4nhs.org.uk

38 Degrees – online campaign organisation https://home.38degrees.org.uk

London Health Emergency – campaigns against NHS privatisation since 1988 https://healthemergency.org.uk

NHS for Sale http://www.nhsforsale.info/

The Doctors Association UK https://www.dauk.org

2. Engage with the NHS – by attending a local CCG board meeting, or a patient participation group at your GP surgery, and ask about members conflicts of interests. Challenge proposed changes to local services on anything other than clinical grounds and ask for a pro-NHS approach. There is a statutory requirement for NHS bodies to publicly consult when a significant change to the service is planned (such as hospital closures) and the NHS constitution gives us a right to be involved in the planning of healthcare services. Find out about local meetings (which are usually open to the public) by searching your local CCG, Trust or local authority webpage, or using your local Healthwatch: http://www.healthwatch.co.uk/find-local-healthwatch

3. Write to your MP and engage with local media. Find out who your MP is here: www.theyworkforyou.com and write a letter to your MP.

4. For NHS staff – support initiatives that improve efficiency in the NHS. COVID-19 has demonstrated that radical changes can take place within the system without months of prior discussion. Encourage flexible/home working for staff with parental or caring responsibilities. Champion electronic prescribing and telemedicine where appropriate for hospital teams as well as GPs. Throw away fax machines and make technology work to improve the service.

5. For NHS Patients – Use the service responsibly. Don't miss appointments. Don't call an ambulance without a clinical need for one because of transport issues. Consider using 111 or a pharmacist for minor ailments rather than your GP or A&E. Don't order repeat medications that you are not intending to use and consider buying over the counter medications where possible. Make healthy lifestyle choices to prevent chronic disease.

Chapter 5

Pandemic

On New Year's Eve 2019, local government authorities in Wuhan, Hubei Province, China released a health alert, announcing clusters of a mysterious pneumonia in their city. Doctors in Wuhan noticed that many of the patients presenting with this new disease had all visited the city's Huanan seafood market before getting ill. Less than a month later the city went into lockdown to control what had grown into an epidemic of the new virus – which of course we now know as COVID-19.

The COVID-19 pandemic is the defining global health crisis of our time. It has reached every continent except Antarctica, and at the time of writing there are 31.6 million cases and 972,000 deaths worldwide, with cases continuing to rise daily, particularly in Africa, Europe and the Americas. The rest of the world watched Wuhan with fascination in January 2020 as the city shut down, oblivious to what was in store – a global lockdown, billions confined to their homes while scientists around the world raced to discover treatments and make a vaccine.

1918 Influenza Pandemic – 'Spanish Flu'

Before we delve into COVID-19 – lets step back 100 years to talk about the last significant pandemic to hit the world. As the Great War was drawing to an end, a new threat emerged that went on to kill three times the number of people claimed by the war. The Spanish Influenza pandemic of 1918-20 took the lives of at least 50-100 million people around the world, striking down healthy young adults in their 20s and 30s. One in three people on earth, or 500 million human beings were infected. More died in a single year, than died in the four years of the Black death (1347-51). Every continent, bar Antartica was affected, and only Australia, who imposed strict quarantine measures, was spared.

It was nicknamed 'Spanish flu' as the first reported cases were in Spain (and famously, one of the first casualties was the King of Spain), but cases emerged simultaneously in pockets across the globe in the spring of 1918. As the war was still ongoing, many countries had imposed media blackouts, which censored reports of the disease, in an attempt to maintain morale. Offended by the slander, war-neutral Spain named the disease 'Naples soldier'. All over the world, people chose names for the pandemic, that placed blame for it elsewhere. In Brazil it was 'German flu' and in Poland, 'Bolshevik disease'. The Persians blamed the British, while the Japanese blamed their sumo wrestlers when it first broke out at a sumo wrestling tournament. Once the pandemic was global, it became necessary to agree on a single name – and since the victors of the great war were calling it Spanish flu, the name stuck.

The UK was hit by the first wave of the disease when troops returned from the trenches in France at the end of the First World War. Today, seasonal influenza is especially risky for the elderly and vulnerable groups with underlying health conditions, but Spanish flu mainly affected young adults, and those above the age of 75 had the lowest death rate of all. The disease swept across the country, spreading at an alarming rate, in a series of waves starting first in Glasgow and reaching London by June 1918. Cases had reduced by August, but then a second wave returned in October, more deadly than the first, followed by a milder third wave in early 1919 - ultimately claiming the lives of 228,000 people in Britain.

A Doctor's Letter From 1918

A letter from a doctor working in US Army Barracks, dated 29 September 1918, was published in the BMJ in 1979 and describes his horror at facing this new disease:

'Camp Devens is near Boston, and has about 50,000 men, or did have before this epidemic broke loose. This epidemic started about four weeks ago, and has developed so rapidly that the camp is demoralised and all ordinary work is held up till it has passed. These men start with what appears to be an ordinary attack of LaGrippe or Influenza, [then] they rapidly develop the most vicious type of pneumonia that has ever been seen. Two hours after admission they have the mahogany spots over the cheek bones, and a few hours later you can begin to see the Cyanosis [blue colour due to lack of oxygen] extending from their ears and spreading all over the face. It is only a matter of hours then until death comes, and it is simply a struggle for air until they suffocate. We have been averaging about 100 deaths per day. There is no doubt in my mind that there is a new mixed infection here, but what I don't know. For several days there were no coffins and the bodies piled up something fierce, and we used to go down to the morgue and look at the boys laid out in long rows. It beats any sight they ever had in France after a battle.

Britain was slow to respond. Worried about hindering the nations war effort, senior medical officer Sir Arthur Newsholme essentially told Britons to 'Keep Calm and Carry On', creating a perfect environment for mass infection. Sir Arthur told The Royal Society of Medicine that 'The relentless needs of warfare justify the risks of spreading infection' and that Britain's major duty was to carry on largely as normal, 'even when risk to health and life is involved'.

Spanish flu was not mentioned as an issue in parliament until October 1918, and without a national health service in place, the response was uncoordinated, with each town relying on its existing resources to cope, with no central government guidance or imposed lockdown. The war effort had diverted over 50 per cent of medical staff to the front lines, meaning that those left to deal with the pandemic were older doctors not in military service, who often became victims to the illness themselves. The concept of a virus was novel in 1918, and medics assumed they were dealing with a bacterial disease, which they named 'Pfeiffer's bacillus'. It was not until 1933 and the invention of the electron microscope, that it was concluded that Spanish flu was caused by a virus. Doctors were helpless against the scourge, as they had no vaccines, no antivirals and no antibiotics (which may have been effective against the secondary bacterial infections that killed many victims in the form of pneumonia). The disease was recognised as being contagious from the start but was only declared notifiable to the authorities once the third wave had struck in 1919. This hampered any attempts at early quarantine measures, since authorities failed to see the pandemic approaching. At the time, healthcare in Britain was provided mainly by local authorities, whose main concern was not health care provision, but operating the Poor Law.

Local authorities gave a variety of advice to the public– some more sensible than others. Self isolation was advised in Hackney, London, while people in Brighton were told 'to give up shaking hands for the present, and give up kissing for all time'. Hundreds of elementary schools around the country were closed, but secondary schools remained open, as did churches, on the grounds that religion would help people through the crisis. Inhaling cool air was a much valued idea, and many isolation hospitals nursed patients outside in the open air. Some reportedly placed patients in soaking wet beds and sprinkled them regularly with cold water, in an attempt to stimulate their immune systems.

The bizarre advice kept coming. 'Eat plenty of porridge' advised the News of the World, and 'wash inside nose with soap and water each night'; 'Clean your teeth regularly' said one government official. Many factories relaxed no smoking rules, believing the smoke would

An open air hospital ward in 1918 https://wellcomecollection.org/works/kjsu8783. (The Royal Hospital, Haslar, England: an open-air tuberculosis ward. Photograph, 1914/1918. Credit: Wellcome Collection. Attribution 4.0 International (CC BY 4.0))

prevent infection, while others started eating raw onions and knocking back shots of whisky. A Scottish doctor made the observation that hardly any of his influenza patients worked at the local jam factory and started prescribing jam and sweets for his patients.

The efforts made in other countries to contain the disease were more robust. In America, public gatherings were banned and schools, churches and cinemas all closed. Masks were distributed and some states banned handshaking. In Spain, passengers travelling by train were sprayed with disinfectant, while Australia kept the disease at bay for some time by imposing quarantine and ensuring any travellers entering the country stayed in isolation. This protocol has been repeated in Australia during the COVID-19 pandemic with good initial results.

Lessons Learned

By the time the pandemic had subsided in 1920, 228,000 people had died in Britain, and up to 100 million worldwide. Britain had been hit hard in the preceding war years – millions were dead or wounded, industry was disrupted and the country was ill-equipped to cope with the pandemic. Letters to newspapers at the time condemned the government's tardiness in demobilising doctors at the front. 'Schemes for checking these terrible visitations need to be thought out and prepared beforehand,' complained the *Hackney Gazette*. While the *Perthshire Advertiser* noted: 'We possess much more stringent laws in regard to the health of animals than to that of human beings.'

Some lessons were learned, however. Authorities realised that blaming an individual for catching a disease was no longer reasonable and public health policy adapted accordingly. Governments around the world embraced socialised medicine in the 1920s. Russia led the way by recognising that the prevention of illness is just as important as curing it and advocated studying the occupational and social conditions which give rise to illness. The collection of health data became more organised and the disease reporting systems which had been lacking in 1918 were established.

In 1919, an international bureau for fighting epidemics was opened in Vienna – a forerunner of The World Health Organisation (WHO) – which was set up in 1948, as a specialised agency of the United

Nations, concerned with International Public Health. WHO began its global influenza surveillance and response system in 1948, aiming to track flu outbreaks across the world and identify possible pandemics – recognising that the control of a pandemic is a social problem, not an individual one. The basic public health measures we saw being carried out across the world to contain COVID-19 (isolating and quarantining; contact tracing; school/workplace closures – so called 'non-pharmaceutical measures') can be regarded as a legacy of the lessons learned from Spanish flu.

Let's return to COVID-19.

What is in a Name?

Naming a disease is a sensitive exercise. When a disease first emerges, naming it creates a semblance of control, but often a name is attributed before scientists have fully grasped the characteristics of the disease – causing problems later. The name first given to 'AIDS' in the 1980s was 'gay-related immune deficiency', which subsequently stigmatised the homosexual community. 'Ebola' was named for the River Ebola in Central Africa where it was first reported, but in 2014 caused an outbreak in West Africa.

The WHO created guidelines in 2015 in attempt to minimise the negative impacts of disease names on trade, travel and animal welfare and to avoid causing offence to any groups of people. Vetoed terms included any geographical locations or cultural references such as 'Spanish flu', 'Japanese encephalitis', 'Legionnaires disease'. Reference to animals or food ('Swine flu') were out, as were any terms that incited fear (using words such as 'fatal' or 'unknown').

On 11 February 2020, the WHO announced that the disease caused by this novel coronavirus would be called Coronavirus disease 2019 or 'COVID-19'. The new coronavirus identified as causing the disease was named 'Severe Acute Respiratory Syndrome Coronavirus 2' (SARS-CoV-2).

What is a Coronavirus?

Coronaviruses are a large family of viruses which includes the common cold, Middle East Respiratory Syndrome (MERS) and Severe

Acute Respiratory Syndrome (SARS). A novel coronavirus, such as COVID-19 is a new strain of coronavirus that has not been previously identified in humans.

Coronaviruses are very common in the world of veterinary medicine – since they affect many domestic animal species (dogs, cats, pigs, poultry to name a few). Bats, birds and rodents are recognised as natural reservoirs – meaning, these species carry the virus, but don't become unwell from it. We know that many disease-causing microbes only infect animals, some only infect humans, and others that can infect both. Most animal coronaviruses such as canine and feline coronaviruses only infect animals and not humans. Coronaviruses have a history of transferring between species. In 2002, SARS was transmitted to humans via civet cats, and in 2012, MERS jumped from dromedary camels to humans. The exact source of COVID-19 is not known for certain, but it is known that it made the jump to humans from an animal source, since the first infections were linked to a live animal market. Human to human transmission then occurred extensively, through respiratory droplet and fomite spread (SARS-CoV-2 has also been detected in blood, faeces and urine).

COVID-19 is made up of a single strand of RNA (Ribonucleic acid), protected by a fatty membrane which is covered in crown-like spikes (which give it its name – corona means crown). The fatty membrane breaks apart in contact with soap – which is why handwashing has been so emphasised. This tiny microbe measures a mere 120 nanometres across – which means you can fit a hundred million viral particles on the head of a pin. The virus is mainly spread through coughing and sneezing. You only need to inhale a few hundred viral particles to become infected.

Genome sequence data from SARS-CoV-2 has been analysed and compared to known coronavirus strains which has determined that the virus is the product of natural evolution – disproving conspiracy theories that the virus was engineered in a laboratory. Scientists identified that the receptor-binding domain (the part of the virus that allows it to enter host cells) has evolved so effectively to bind onto human cells that this could only be a result of natural selection rather than genetic engineering. Furthermore, they found that the molecular structure of SARS-CoV-2 resembled that of related viruses in bats and pangolins, suggesting the virus evolved to its current state in the animal host (probably bats) and jumped to humans. There are no documented cases of direct bat–human transmission, which suggests an intermediate host is likely to be involved (probably Malayan pangolins). At present, until more evidence is available, these scenarios are theoretical.

Clinical Features

By now, everyone is aware of the key symptoms of COVID-19 (table 5.1) As early as January 2020, *The Lancet* published the first clinical description. Many patients appeared to have a mild illness and a rapid recovery, but around 20 per cent were not so fortunate and developed severe symptoms. Cough and fever were the commonest presenting symptoms, along with muscle aches and fatigue. Those developing severe illness typically developed shortness of breath around a week after the initial symptoms and pneumonia which can progress quickly to acute respiratory distress syndrome. In the most severe cases, the infection triggered their immune systems to release a flood of immune cells known as a cytokine storm, which attacked the healthy tissues they should be protecting. Patients developed multiple organ failure, blood clots and secondary infections. The Chinese doctors were clearly concerned back in January, stressing that no treatment existed for the 'serious, sometimes fatal pneumonia' that developed, other than supportive treatment from a ventilator on an intensive care unit. They were clear in their reports, that this new coronavirus had 'pandemic potential' as the number of deaths from it was rising quickly.

Like many viral illnesses, some people can have the virus but display no symptoms (asymptomatic). Symptoms typically appear 2-14 days after exposure to the virus – 5 days on average, which is why contacts of a person with the disease are asked to quarantine for 14 days. During this timescale, known as the incubation period, people can be infectious before they develop any symptoms, and can remain infectious for up to 10 days – sometimes longer. The more severe the infection, the higher the viral load, and the longer a patient will continue to shed virus and remain infectious. The WHO warned on 16th March that quarantine measures should be extended for another 14 days after recovering from symptoms of COVID-19, as people may still be contagious. In the UK, people with symptoms were advised to isolate for 7 days, and to only extend this period if they continued to have a fever, which is at odds with guidance from the WHO and other countries.

Table 5.1. Symptoms of COVID-19 (WHO https://www.who.int/health-topics/coronavirus#tab=tab_3)

Most Common Symptoms	Less Common Symptoms	Serious Symptoms
Fever Cough Fatigue	Sore Throat Loss of taste/smell Headache Muscle aches Diarrhoea Conjunctivitis Skin changes (rash; discolouration of fingers/toes)	Difficulty breathing/Shortness of breath Chest pain Loss of speech/movement

COVID-19 – A Timeline

31 Dec 2019
A cluster of cases of pneumonia 'of an unknown cause' are reported to the World Health Organisation by Chinese authorities. The cases were identified on 21st December 2019 in Wuhan, Hubei Province, China. A novel coronavirus is eventually identified.

2 Jan 2020
Central Hospital of Wuhan bans its staff from discussing the disease publicly.

10 Jan 2020
WHO issue guidance to all countries on how to detect, test and manage potential cases based on experience with SARS, MERS and current knowledge of the virus.

11 Jan 2020
The first known death from the virus is reported by Chinese state media – a 61-year-old man who was a regular customer at the market in Wuhan where the virus is believed to have originated. The Wuhan health authority report that those diagnosed with the virus are mainly vendors and purchasers at the city's Huanan Seafood Wholesale Market, which was shut down on 1st Jan 2020. To date, they say, no medical staff are infected with no clear evidence of human-to-human transmission found.

12 Jan 2020
China publicly share the genetic sequence of COVID-19.

13 Jan 2020

The first recorded case of COVID-19 outside of China is reported in Thailand in a traveller who had arrived from Wuhan.

20-22 Jan 2020

Human–human transmission is confirmed. The first case in the United States is confirmed and Public Health England move the risk level to the British public from 'very low' to 'low'.

23 Jan 2020

The cities of Wuhan, Xiantao and Chibi in Hubei province (a total of 56 million people) are quarantined as air and rail departures are suspended. The Chinese Railway administration show that almost 100,000 people had already departed from Wuhan train station before the lockdown. At this point, seventeen deaths have been reported and construction begins in Wuhan for a specialist emergency hospital (which opens on 3 Feb).

25 Jan 2020

The UK Foreign and Commonwealth Office advises against all travel to China's Hubei Province.

26 Jan 2020

Chinese New Year Celebrations take place in central London as thousands gather in Chinatown to celebrate the Year of the Rat. The WHO reports 2,014 cases globally at this point, twenty-nine of these outside of China, and fifty-six deaths.

28 Jan 2020

The WHO Director General travels to Beijing to learn more about China's response to the outbreak. The UK Foreign and Commonwealth Office update their guidance advising against travel to all of mainland China.

29 Jan 2020

The UK's first two patients test positive for COVID-19 – two Chinese nationals from the same family staying at a hotel in York. Britons evacuated from Wuhan arrive in the UK and are quarantined for 14 days at Arrowe Park hospital in Merseyside. British Airways suspends all flights to and from Mainland China.

30 Jan 2020
WHO declares a Public Health Emergency of International Concern (PHEIC), reporting 7,818 total confirmed cases worldwide-the majority in China, with eighty-two cases reported in eighteen other countries. Declaring a PHEIC is a big deal, and means the disease poses a public health risk through international spread and requires a coordinated international response to control it.

3 Feb 2020
The *Diamond Princess* cruise ship is quarantined in Yokohama, Japan, after Japanese authorities are notified of a symptomatic passenger who departed the ship in Hong Kong earlier in the cruise. Two days later, all 3,711 people on board are quarantined. Among these, 712 tested positive for COVID-19. Of these, 331 (46.5%) were asymptomatic at the time of testing. Among the 381 patients with symptoms, 37 required intensive care (9.7%) and 9 died (1.3%).

7 Feb 2020
Dr Li Wenliang, one of the first to raise concerns about COVID-19 in China dies of the virus. He had been reprimanded by authorities in January and made to denounce his warnings about the disease as unfounded. Hong Kong introduces prison sentences for anyone breaking quarantine rules.

11 Feb 2020
WHO announces that SARS-CoV-2 (the new coronavirus identified as causing the disease) will be called COVID-19. 'Covi' for coronavirus, 'D' for disease and '19' for the year it was first identified, 2019. At this point, there are 43,103 cases globally (2,560 new), 1,017 deaths in China (108 new), one death outside of China (first death outside China confirmed in the Philippines). Nine cases have been confirmed in the UK.

14 Feb 2020
Egypt confirms the first recorded case on the African continent. Meanwhile, China is reviewing its trade and consumption of wildlife, which has been identified as a probable source of the outbreak.

19 Feb 2020
Iran confirmed its first two deaths from the disease, hours after confirming its first cases. Six days later, the country emerges as a second focus point for the virus with ninety-five cases and fifteen deaths.

20 Feb 2020

South Korea reports its first death from coronavirus and immediately shuts down thousands of kindergartens, nursing homes and community centres.

23 Feb 2020

Italy sees a surge in cases (150) and ten towns in Lombardy are locked down.

24 Feb 2020

President Trump in the USA asks congress for $1.25 billion for coronavirus response. At this point the country has thirty-five confirmed cases and no deaths. In the UK, minutes from SAGE recommend 'no discharges (from hospital) to care or residential homes'. This did not happen, which in retrospect was a mistake.

25 Feb 2020

UK government guidance advised that travellers returning from Hubei, Iran and South Korea should self-isolate on return home, even if they are asymptomatic. Guidance is issued to care homes in the UK with no restrictions on visits, stating it was 'very unlikely that people receiving care in a care home or the community will become infected'. Another mistake.

26 Feb 2020

The virus reaches Latin America, as Brazilian Health officials report that a man from Sao Paulo tests positive after returning from Italy.

28 Feb 2020

UK authorities confirm the first case of the illness passed on inside the country. The first Briton to die of COVID-19 is confirmed by Japanese authorities – a passenger from the *Diamond Princess* cruise ship. 800 people are now infected in Italy, and Sub-Saharan Africa records its first infection.

29 Feb 2020

The US records its first coronavirus death and announces travel restrictions for Italy, South Korea and Iran. In the UK, twenty-three cases have been confirmed after 10,483 people have been tested. Approximately 442,675 calls are made to NHS 111 in the last week of February.

2 March 2020
The government holds a COBRA meeting to discuss its response to
the virus.

4 March 2020
The biggest surge in cases to date is announced in the UK as thirty-four
new cases bring the total to eighty-seven.

6 March 2020
Prime Minister Boris Johnson announces £46 million in funding
towards COVID-19 research.

8 March 2020
Saudi Arabia imposes lockdown and suspension of schools and
universities after their first case is announced on 5 March.

9 March 2020
The UK Foreign and Commonwealth Office advises against travel to
Italy, while the FTSE 100 drops by more than 8 per cent - its largest
fall since 2008. Three days later it drops by over 10 per cent. The
'Spirit of Shankley', a Liverpool supporters' group raises concerns
about the arrival of up to 3,000 football fans from Madrid ahead of
the forthcoming Liverpool vs Athletico Madrid match two days later.
A council-chaired safety meeting allows the game to go ahead (Spain
has 589 cases at this point – many in Madrid – and declared a 'state of
alarm' four days later).

11 March 2020
The WHO declares the virus a pandemic, as stock markets plunge
and the US bans all travel from Europe (other than the UK) for 30
days. Chancellor Rishi Sunak announces a £30billion package of
emergency support to help the UK cope with coronavirus. The Bank
of England cuts it baseline interest rate to 0.25 per cent – the lowest
level in history (this later drops even lower to 0.1 per cent by the end
of the month).

12 March 2020
Public Health England stops performing contact tracing due to the
wide spread of the infection in the community. The previous advice
for returning travellers is scrapped, with travellers following the same

advice as the rest of the population (which is that anyone with a new continuous cough or fever should self-isolate for seven days.) Sir Patrick Vallance, Chief Scientific Advisor, says the UK is four weeks behind Italy (who at this point has 15,000 cases and more than 100 deaths, compared to the UK's 596 cases and 10 deaths). In reality, the UK reported 1,000 deaths just 16 days later on 28th March. Schools are asked to cancel trips overseas and those over 70 are advised to avoid cruises.

13 March 2020
A multitude of UK sporting events announce their postponement including the Premier League season and the London Marathon, whilst the Cheltenham Gold Cup goes ahead at Cheltenham racecourse attracting an attendance of 251,684.

14 March 2020
The UK government's 'herd immunity' strategy generates controversy, as the number of UK cases rises to 1,140, with twenty-one deaths. UK retailers request customers avoid panic buying, as supermarkets start to sell out of toilet paper, hand gel and pasta.

15 March 2020
The FCO advises against travel to Spain and the USA. Daily televised Government press conferences begin in the UK. Boris Johnson (as PM) or Matt Hancock (Minster for Health) are typically flanked by Professor Chris Whitty (Chief Medical Officer for England) and Sir Patrick Vallance (Chief Scientific Advisor).

16 March 2020
Lockdowns begin around the world to slow the spread of the virus (in Venezuela, Ecuador and Peru. Colombia and Costa Rica Close their borders). In the UK, Boris Johnson encourages Brits to work from home where possible and avoid pubs and restaurants (which remain open) and all non-essential travel. 1,543 cases have been confirmed in the UK, with fifty-five deaths, although actual numbers of those infected is believed to be closer to 10,000. It is unclear why we do not use our Island advantage and close our sea, air and land borders. Businesses are asked to support the supply of ventilators in the UK.

17 March 2020

France imposed a nationwide lockdown as they report 6,500 cases and 140 deaths

In the UK, the biggest package of emergency state support for businesses in announced since the 2008 financial crash, in the form of £330 billion of government backed loans and £20 billion in tax cuts and grants for companies facing collapse. NHS England announces that all elective operations with be postponed from April to free up 30,000 beds to fight COVID-19. A £3.2 million support package is made available by the UK government to support rough sleepers into accommodation during the pandemic.

18 March 2020

The UK government announces that all schools will close from 20 March and all exams are cancelled.

19 March 2020

The GMC grant emergency registration to 15,000 doctors who had given up their registration in the last three years, including thousands of recently retired doctors who also join the efforts against the pandemic. Revalidation checks are placed on hold during the pandemic. New Zealand closes its borders and imposes two weeks supervised quarantine on any New Zealanders returning from overseas. China reports zero local infections for the first time.

My NHS Story – Covid Diaries

Dr Jenny Abthorpe (BSc MBBS FRCA MRCP PGCert Clin Ed FHEA FFICM MAcadME) worked in London as a Registrar in Intensive Care Medicine and Anaesthesia as the pandemic broke. She documented her experiences in a series of diary entries for family and friends, which have been shared throughout the timeline.

'In January 2020, I was a dual trainee in Intensive Care Medicine and Anaesthesia with only six months left before I gained my Certificate of Completion of Training (CCT). I had recently taken a year of maternity leave and returned to my role as an ST7 doctor in Critical Care at King's College Hospital in London. I felt the usual nerves in returning after a year out, but quickly settled back in, enjoying the new challenge of balancing work with a 13-month old. Little did I know about the challenges ahead.

'I first heard about COVID-19 at the end of January. Like most people, it seemed a distant threat and one that held little concern for those of us in the UK. As things progressed, I remember feeling shocked at the accounts coming out of China and immense sympathy for both the medical professional dealing with the outbreak and the residents of Wuhan. I never imagined that only six weeks later I would be witnessing the start of the pandemic in London.

'I was attending a Critical Care ultrasound course in Portsmouth on Friday 28th February, when I heard the news that the first COVID-19 transmission within the UK had been confirmed. The general feeling among the attendees on the course was that a UK outbreak was inevitable but when and how bad, no one knew.

'Early March heralded the wave of the pandemic in Lombardy, Italy. Italian intensivists and their colleagues sounded the alarm loud and clear. COVID-19 was coming to the UK and we needed to heed their warnings and prepare. Behind the scenes at King's, major incident planning began in earnest. The bronze, silver and gold command teams began to meet regularly to discuss and plan the raft of changes that would need to be implemented as the pandemic hit. Our Emergency Department (ED) had already responded to the imminent threat of COVID-19 and had instigated changes a few weeks before. Frontline staff were trained in donning and doffing personal protective equipment (PPE) and were fit tested for the special masks required for dealing with respiratory infectious diseases. Our department held teaching sessions on COVID-19, researching and disseminating as much up to date information as possible to help us prepare. We wrote, designed and implemented simulation training to prepare for intubating and transferring COVID-19 patients. There was an intense atmosphere of purpose, focus and anticipation mixed with nerves. It was like preparing for battle but against an unknown enemy. COVID-19 was a novel disease and for the first time for all of us, from the most senior to the most junior, we were all as inexperienced as each other. But this is what we were trained to do, and we were ready.

'Our index case was identified and admitted to our first receiving intensive care unit (ICU) on Tuesday 10 March. I was based on the ICU

An empty platform at rush hour – Clapham Junction (one of Britain's busiest stations), 24 March 2020 17:50

that day and remember thinking 'Here we go.' It was almost a relief that we could finally get on with getting to know this new adversary.

'The following are extracts from a diary I wrote for family, friends and colleagues during the pandemic. I found it a very cathartic process during what was an incredibly busy and stressful time. I wrote much of it sat on a train or platform while on my way to and from work, trying to process and make sense of what was happening.'

19 March 2020

I know a lot of doctors are very scared. For themselves and their families. Me too. I was on-call yesterday and spent nearly all of it with COVID-19 positive patients. Some needed intubation and ICU. Some were doing fine and just needed reassurance and good ward care. Some were deteriorating but sadly not appropriate for ICU and were being managed as end-of-life patients. They were from all ethnic backgrounds with ages ranging from 20 to 90, from all walk of life and religions. Some were fit and well usually, others had significant co-morbidities.

None of them had travel or contact history. I suspect all of them had contracted it from family and friends rather than random strangers. What unified them is that they and their families were scared and bewildered.

On ICU it's pretty calm and controlled at the moment. Our beds are steadily being filled but we have a comprehensive plan to expand our capacity to 200% plus. I've no doubt we're only at the beginning of the initial wave. The wards, however are carnage. Nurses refusing to enter rooms of COVID-19 positive patients. Physiotherapists not wanting to attend. People using inappropriate PPE as they don't trust surgical masks and Public Health England guidance. Simple infection control measures being forgotten. General fear and confusion, while the patients lie in their beds just needing good nursing and medical care, and their families sit by their bedside feeling helpless.

Doctors from any specialty can lead the response on the wards (or in the community). Any one of us can hold the hand of a scared patient, talk to a family, reassure, manage end of life care and support and educate the nurses. Let's not turn COVID-19 patients into the Lepers of the medieval ages or the HIV patients of the '80s. Please ... it's ok to be scared. Follow PPE guidelines, hand hygiene and simple infection control measures. But remember, as scared as we are, our patients and colleagues look to us for guidance and reassurance. Let's step up as a profession and be the beacon of light during what may be a very dark time.

Stay safe. Be strong. Be kind

20 March 2020

Social venues throughout the UK are ordered to close, while the government promises to pay up to 80 per cent of wages for workers being laid off. Northwick Park Hospital in North London announces a 'critical incident' due to a surge in patients with COVID-19. Singapore is the first country to launch a COVID-19 contact tracing app, releasing 'Trace Together', which records encounters with other app users by Bluetooth, facilitating the contact tracing process should a user become ill.

21 March 2020

NHS England block books almost all of the country's private hospital facilities in preparation to fight COVID-19.

22 March 2020

5,600 former nurses re-register with the Nursing and Midwifery Council to offer their services during the pandemic. At the start of the year, more than one in ten nursing posts were vacant.

23 March 2020
The UK goes into lockdown. Boris Johnson announces that people should only leave the house to buy food, to exercise once a day or to go to work if it is impossible to work from home. The Coronavirus Act is passed a few days later (The Health Protection (Coronavirus restrictions) (England) Regulations 2020), giving powers to the police to fine citizens who do not comply with these measures. Australia also goes into lockdown.

24 March 2020
UK Health Secretary Matt Hancock announces that a temporary hospital will be opened at the ExCel London to provide extra critical care capacity – to be called the NHS Nightingale Hospital. He also announces that 5,500 final year medical students will join the workforce early alongside student nurses and midwives.

25 March 2020
NHS Staff begin to die from COVID-19. The first two working NHS doctors die on the same day, GP Dr Habib Zaidi and Surgeon Dr Adil El Tayar.

Routine dental care is suspended in England, Prince Charles tests positive for COVID-19 and police are given powers to use 'reasonable force' to enforce lockdown regulations. Elsewhere, the Tokyo Olympics are postponed. India locks down its 1.3 billion residents after recording 536 cases. Brazilian President Jair Bolsonaro objects to coronavirus measures being taken in his country, leading to local officials taking action themselves. The UN launched a $2 billion global humanitarian response plan to fight COVID-19 in some of the world's most vulnerable countries.

Memorial of Health and Social Care Workers

A digital tribute was set up by 'Nursing Notes' as a memorial to the members of staff who died during the COVID-19 Pandemic. They also pledged to plant a tree for every life lost. At the time of writing, at least 620 healthcare workers have died from COVID-19. The memorial can be accessed: https://nursingnotes.co.uk/COVID-19-memorial/#

26 March 2020

The weekly 'Clap for Our Carers' begins as Brits across the UK stand on their doorsteps at 8pm every Thursday to clap and cheer for the NHS staff working throughout the pandemic. Founded by Annemarie Plas, a Dutch expatriate living in London, who had seen a similar event in the Netherlands, Italy and Spain, the movement went on every Thursday through lockdown until 28th May 2020, with appreciation extending to all keyworkers. An annual Clap for Our Carers Day is planned for the last Thursday of March each year moving forward.

27 March 2020

Prime Minister Boris Johnson and Health Secretary Matt Hancock test positive for COVID-19. Johnson is later admitted to an intensive care unit in early April. At a press conference three weeks earlier, Johnson told reporters he was still shaking hands, despite advice from the WHO not to. 'I was at a hospital the other night where I think there were actually a few coronavirus patients and I shook hands with everybody,' he said. Chris Whitty, the England's Chief Medical Officer also self isolates after experiencing symptoms. Leon Restaurants starts the 'Feed NHS' project to deliver free meals to NHS critical care staff in London.

My NHS Story – Dr Jenny Abthorpe – Covid Diaries

27 March 2020
Today I went to work.

Ate my breakfast on the empty train. Watched the beautiful frosty scenery go past. Thought about the patients I'd seen recently in the ED who needed ICU and hoped they had survived another night. I walked past the warning signs at the hospital entrance and then those on the doors to the ICU. I'm used to them now.

I changed into my scrubs, donned my mask and sat in handover for an update on each patient. Handover now takes over an hour as we have a full ICU. Forty-six patients in critical care. An increase of twenty-eight in a week. Age range 28-70. Most with minor underlying medical problems.

I'm assigned my four patients and don full PPE to enter the 'risk' zone to briefly examine each patient. Switching gloves and washing hands between each case. I touch base with each nurse. Do they need anything? Any concerns? Are they ok? And thank each of them for their incredible work. Every nurse is in full PPE for their entire shift except breaks. They are superhuman.

We're beginning to know this silent enemy. The virus. Patterns are emerging. But it's frustrating and slow. Those patients that are doing less well, we feel at a loss to know how to halt their decline. We focus on the best evidence-based practice and gather advice from regional, national and international critical care networks. We lost some patients this week and that's been tough. Some patients have been transferred out for ECMO (extracorporeal membrane oxygenation-a form of life support). But we've also had successes. Patients have been liberated from their ventilators successfully, have been discharged from ICU and are doing well. Significant milestones which have boosted morale.

We snatch a few minutes for lunch. So grateful for the delicious food being donated by local restaurants. A definite highlight of the day! The afternoons are hectic. Stabilising sick patients. Proning (positioning patients face down rather than on their back) those who need escalating treatment for refractory hypoxia. Dealing with new admissions. There's now a sense of urgency and feeling of pressure. But we know what we need to do and pull together as a team. Nurses are being redeployed from all over the hospital to assist us. Our anaesthetic colleagues are supporting us too. Critical care is expanding into new areas of the hospital with the contingency plan to achieve 300+ beds.

A new admission arrives at 6pm. He deteriorated on the ward and needs intubation. They're too busy to perform it there so bring him to us. He sits there trembling with fear. Wide-eyed as he stares around him. I don my PPE and go to reassure him. He's exhausted. I drift him off to sleep, reassuring him that I will see him soon. He will be fine and we will take good care of him. He will never be alone, with a nurse always watching over him. He holds my hand and says 'See you in the morning ... thank you doctor.' My heart breaks a little. Half an hour later he is stable and settled. I put my hand on his forehead and whisper 'Please do well'. A small plea.

I sit on the train home, it is so quiet and empty. London is still. Londoners have finally listened. And I feel relief.

Its 22:00 and now I'm home. Showered and clean. Sat on the sofa with my husband. After sneaking into the nursery to stroke my little one's head. Another day over. A precious weekend off and then back again...

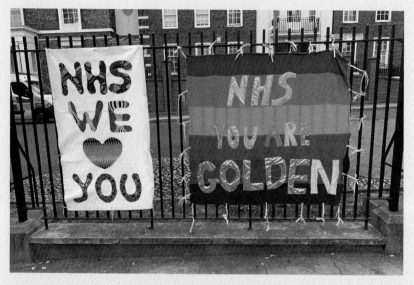

Thank you NHS-Signs outside Kings Hospital.

30 March 2020
UK Foreign Secretary Dominic Raab announces the government will spend £75 million on charter flights to repatriate 300,000 Britons stranded abroad due to COVID-19.

31 March 2020
At the end of March, Spain, Italy and the USA report more cases than China. More than 10,000 people are hospitalised in the UK with COVID-19 and a UK daily death toll of 381 takes the total number of deaths to 1,789.

1 April 2020
UK Minister Michael Gove says a shortage of reagents needed to perform COVID-19 testing means it is not possible to screen the entire

NHS workforce of 1.2 million people. 2,000 NHS staff have been tested. The Chemical Industries Association go on to contradict this statement, stating that there is not a shortage.

2 April 2020

The worldwide total number of cases passes one million. The UK government writes off £13.4 billion of historic debts across the NHS to give trusts financial support during the pandemic and beyond. Guidance is issued by DHSC for care homes, only now advising family and friends not to visit except in exceptional circumstances such as at the end of life.

3 April 2020

NHS Nightingale Hospital London is opened by the Prince of Wales (via video). Designed to provide care for up to 500 patients requiring intensive care treatment who have already been intubated and ventilated, it is built in nine days with the help of army engineers, contractors and NHS staff. Further hospitals are planned in Manchester, Birmingham, Bristol and Harrogate to provide hundreds of extra beds should local services need them during the peak of the pandemic.

My NHS Story – Dr Jenny Abthorpe – Covid Diaries

3 April

Today I went to work. Cycled down the country lanes to the train station. And stopped briefly to appreciate the dawn chorus, such a beautiful sound. Nature giving me an uplifting, almost reassuring accompaniment to the start of my day. 'You can do this,' it sings. The station is deserted. I feel like a lone warrior as I step onto the train.

It has been a difficult week on our ICU. We had six patients die. I can't remember ever losing this many in a week. And I can't stop thinking about the relative of one of the patients who died. An 81-year-old mother, phoning each day to enquire about her son. Her tremulous frail voice and the sound of relief as I update her that he is doing ok. I feel physical pain as I think of the phone-call made to her the day before. That her son has died. And the fact that she wasn't able to get to the hospital in time.

As I near the hospital, I join the army of NHS workers starting their day. And feel a sense of pride and belonging. The ICU is incredibly busy now. The number of COVID-19 patients requiring critical care is rising swiftly. Our unit is full again with thirty patients, having received six new admissions overnight.

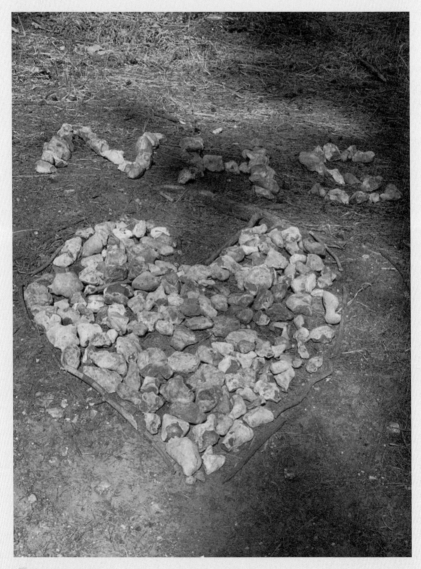

NHS Stone Heart.

The handover is quick and efficient. The night team of two doctors look exhausted. We give them a round of applause to send them on their way home. Heroes.

COVID-19 patients have now filled a 2nd 15-bedded ICU on site. And a 10-bedded unit, created in a former HDU area, is also full. There are now thirty-four beds in theatre recovery which are slowly being filled. PICU are taking non-COVID adult patients. Two other ICUs are increasing their bed capacity in preparation for the surge. Staff are being redeployed from around the hospital to join the ranks of critical care staff. And we are so grateful to them. The morale of the department is high with support coming from every department and staff level.

The day goes by in a blur. Some patients are early on in their illness and need stabilising, life-saving care being instituted. Others are static in their progress and we analyse their numbers and clinical picture, trying to move them forward. Some are getting better and are nearing discharge. We have had some great successes. A colleague and I perform a tracheostomy in a patient who has recovered but is weak and needs slow weaning from the ventilator. But we are delighted that he has got this far.

End of shift. An hour train ride and then cycle home. Two hours later I am home and showered. Just in time to cuddle my little one and read her favourite bedtime story 'Spot Says Goodnight'. Precious moments.

It is getting harder to switch off from work. Sleep is slow to come and nights are restless. COVID-19 fills my thoughts. But a bit of mindless TV and debrief with my husband puts those thoughts to rest for now. Bedtime. Ready for my on-call night shift tomorrow.

4 April 2020
UK road traffic levels are reported to have fallen by 73 per cent since lockdown began, their lowest levels since 1955.

5 April 2020
Scotland's Chief Medical Officer Catherine Calderwood resigns from her position after going against her own 'Stay at home' advice and is pictured visiting her second home. Boris Johnson is admitted to hospital.

6 April 2020
Boris Johnson is taken into intensive care. The UK COVID-19 death toll exceeds 5,000, with almost 52,000 reported cases.

8 April 2020
Thought to be the peak of the pandemic, with the highest number of daily deaths recorded (over 1000) – this number starts to fall after this date

9 April 2020
China intensifies screening of asymptomatic COVID-19 cases in an attempt to prevent a second wave of infection.

10 April 2020
The number of confirmed deaths worldwide passes 100,000. The UK government announces that lockdown measures are having some impact as case numbers fall in London. Further north, case numbers continue to rise in Yorkshire and the North East.

11 April 2020
Personal Protective Equipment (PPE) and the lack of it has remained a concern for frontline workers throughout the pandemic, with many improvising their own due to short supplies. UK Home Secretary Priti Patel says 'sorry if people feel there have been failings' in providing kit.

12 April 2020
The number of people in the UK who died in hospital of COVID-19 passes 10,000. Boris Johnson is discharged from hospital.

13 April 2020
China tackles a resurgence of the virus as the number of daily infections rises to 108, the highest in six weeks. 90 per cent of cases come from abroad.

14 April 2020
Spain eases some lockdown restrictions. Mobile phone operators report more than twenty arson attacks on mobile phone masts in the UK. The surge in attacks are thought to be caused by conspiracy theories which falsely claim that 5G networks have caused COVID-19.

My NHS Story – Dr Jenny Abthorpe – Covid Diaries

April 14 2020
This week I went to work and completed a set of night shifts like no other I have experienced before.

I arrived for each of my shifts with a sense of foreboding, very aware that the peak of the pandemic is coming ever closer and worried about what each shift will bring. At the start of each shift, I join the critical outreach team for their handover, as the day team go through each of the patients on the outreach list. It is staggering. Approximately 20-40 patients on the list each night. All COVID-19 positive or suspected. And all on 60 per cent oxygen or more. Those on less get discharged from the list! The new 'normal'

We are proning awake patients on the ward. Some patients are getting CPAP (Continuous positive airway pressure – a form of breathing support for those who can breathe themselves but need help). Some are on 15 litres of oxygen, unable to be weaned down. All are being reviewed regularly during the day by the outreach team led by an ICU consultant. Many patients are sick but stable, some improving and a few give us cause for concern. The night team will work tirelessly all night to make sure that every patient is seen and safe. Over the week, 1-2 deteriorating patients are intubated each night and taken to one of the ICUs.

The bleep I hold is the outward facing bleep and covers referrals from ED – all critically ill medical and surgical patients, all trauma calls and cardiac arrests. I also provide support and advice to any of the residents and Specialist Registrars on the units. And the number of units has expanded over the past weeks with ventilated patients in newly designated critical care areas. As of last week, there is also a resident ICU consultant on call, absolute godsend!

Multiple ED referrals are received throughout each night. Majority are suspected COVID-19 patients and profoundly hypoxic (low in oxygen). The biggest challenge is trying to provide patient-centred care when each patient presenting is identical to each other – hypertensive +\- diabetic +\- raised BMI with cough, fever, hypoxia and respiratory distress. They blur into one. But what strikes me is that most are surprisingly calm. There is little surprise when I tell them that we think they have coronavirus and may need to go on a ventilator. Just quiet acceptance. I make many phone calls to families from ED, *hating the thought of them seeing their relative taken away and not hearing any news. I update them on their relative's progress and gain vital information on their loved one's baseline. Information that has important bearing on their treatment escalation. The emotion down the phone is tangible. But the families are so grateful for any news and grateful that we will take them to ICU if needed. Not all need it now, but most do.*

The family of an 80-year-old man particularly resonates. His wife tells me she is a retired nurse of thirty-five years. In between sobs, she expresses her gratitude for the care we are giving. I feel so choked up, I can barely say anything. It's humbling. I promise her I will deliver a message to him. And I do. We hold hands for a moment as I whisper the words she told me to tell him. He nods and smiles. He tells me he does not want to come to ICU. Two days later, he passes away on the ward, having seen his family for the final time.

But the referrals are not just COVID-19 related. We have a code red HEMS (Helicopter emergency medical service) trauma come in. A young man who has jumped from a significant height, his injuries are devastating. Two patients are referred with low GCS (unconscious) who we discover have had catastrophic brain haemorrhages. One dies in ED with their family around them, the other goes to the ICU for prognostication and possible organ donation. Four out-of-hospital cardiac arrests come in, three of whom survive with potential for full recovery. One recreational drug overdose. A urosepsis with septic shock and multi-organ failure. The ED team and phenomenal Advanced Critical Care Practitioners (ACCPs) provide fantastic support. Working with me to stabilise each patient, keeping me fed and watered throughout the nights with their usual high-end banter, ensuring all of our morale is kept high. It is not very busy in Resus but those that come in are super sick. It is time-consuming and intense.

But I feel relief, all of these cases are ICU bread and butter. But the difference is, they may all have COVID-19, so it's all done wearing PPE. For hours on end. There are huge communication challenges. It's distracting. The glare from the visors makes putting in endotracheal tubes and lines challenging. And having to wear sterile gowns, gloves etc over the PPE makes it hot and sweaty work. There are times I want to scream and just rip the mask off. My nose is bruised, my cheeks sore. Even when I am finally at home, lying in bed, trying to sleep ... I still feel the sensation of a mask on my face.

Dr Abthorpe in full PPE.

And then there are the ICUs. The doctors and nurses on each unit work tirelessly all night. So many sick patients. The consultant and I attend many emergencies on the Covid units throughout the nights. A number of cardiac arrests. Some ventilator emergencies. We lose patients. The phone calls to the relatives are like a kick in the stomach. The grief down the phone is heartbreaking and I struggle to hold it in myself, voice breaking as I tell another family, 'I'm so sorry.' It feels so inadequate.

But there are many getting better, including my patient from the other week. He's doing really well and I'm so relieved. Each patient that beats this terrible disease needs to be remembered and celebrated. As do those who sadly lose their battle.

The nurses in particular are struggling. They feel like they are fighting fires all the time and not able to give the standard of care they usually do. But what they are achieving is superhuman. And still they keep going. We all do. The incredible anaesthetists now part of the ICU family, the unflappable and highly skilled ACCPs, the fantastic ED doctors, the superb and awe-inspiring medical doctors on the wards, the wonderful ward nurses, the doctors and nurses from other specialties now deployed to the critical cares, the Health Care Assistants and cleaners, the GPs, physiotherapists, pharmacists, mortuary workers, the bereavement office … we all keep going. Because we are the NHS. Because our patients and country need us. And in the future we will say, 'we were there', but who knows what the toll on us will be….

And now I'm home. Enjoying a long Easter bank holiday. Feeling both blessed and guilty for being off. Resting and recuperating for the week ahead.

The ICU Team at Kings.

15 April 2020

Confirmed COVID-19 infections passes 2 million worldwide. Donald Trump, whose own handling of the pandemic is questionable, cuts WHO funding claiming the organisation 'failed in its basic duty' in its response to COVID-19. The US is the largest single funder of WHO. Bill Gates, the second largest, criticised Trumps decision by tweeting: 'Halting funding for the WHO during a world health crisis is as dangerous as it sounds. Their work is slowing the spread of COVID-19 and if that work is stopped no other organization can replace them.'

In the UK, concerns are raised that the official death toll for COVID-19 only accounts for those who died in hospital. Testing begins in care homes and for patients being discharged from hospital. The Office for National Statistics indicates that more than 16,000 deaths were recorded in the week ending 3 April – 6,000 higher than the average for that time of year.

16 April 2020
Tom Moore, a 99-year-old war veteran raises over £25 million for NHS Charities Together by completing 100 laps of his garden. The NHS Nightingale Hospital Birmingham is opened (remotely) by Prince William.

17 April 2020
The WHO emphasises that there is no evidence to prove whether someone who has recovered from COVID-19 is immune from the disease. Death registrations in the UK are at 207 per cent of the five-year average this week, with 21,805 deaths registered – COVID-19 is mentioned in 8,730 of these.

18 April 2020
The UK government briefing reports that the virus appears to have a 'disproportionate impact' on Black Asian and Minority Ethnic communities and Public Health England is asked to investigate. Care England, the UKs largest care home representative body estimates that up to 7,500 care home residents may have died due to COVID-19 compared to the official figure of 1,400.

My NHS Story – Dr Jenny Abthorpe – Covid Diaries

19 April
This week I completed a 2nd set of night shifts. My 2nd in two weeks. My first two nights shifts were locum shifts covering for colleagues off sick, providing senior cover on some of the main ICUs. My second two night shifts were covering the outward facing bleep taking emergency referrals from ED.

My goodness what a difference a week makes.
This week, there was a noticeable drop in numbers of COVID-19 patients presenting to our hospital and a significant downtrend in those needing ICU, although there still are patients being admitted. ED was scarily quiet.

I reflect on my night shift on Tuesday 7th April, one of the worst I have ever done, marked forever in my mind. There was a point that night that I had a moment of panic, thinking that if things got much worse, we would not be able to cope. In hindsight, what we were experiencing that week was the peak of the pandemic. And we coped and got through it.

Between 27th February and 15th April, a six-week timeframe, my hospital had dealt with around 2,000 COVID-19 admissions. 243 admitted to critical care beds (not all of these to the ICUs). 1,210 patients have been discharged alive, sixty-four from critical care. Phenomenal numbers.

My first night was on my usual base unit. It has been receiving COVID-19 patients since day one of the pandemic. Staffed by battle-fatigued nurses and doctors, still deep in the fight against the disease. Morale remains high but it is clear that the past five weeks have taken their toll on everyone. Particularly as we are now caring for more healthcare workers, struck down in the line of duty. It is incredibly sobering.

After handover, we allocate patients and get to work. Reviewing and assessing each patient to ensure they have a smooth night and that they are reaching the daily targets set by the day team.

But nothing goes as planned. COVID-19 is an unpredictable disease but does seem to have a temporal element. Late afternoon and the night are common times for patients to deteriorate usually coinciding with high spikes in fever. In a few cases, even as high as 42C.

With the spike in temperature, oxygen consumption/demand dramatically rises, but is unable to be matched by its delivery through damaged and inflamed lungs, and manifests as a significant drop in oxygen levels. A number of patients require proning to improve oxygen delivery, a procedure that is high risk and labour intensive particularly at night. In other patients, proning does not work, and all we can do is support their organs, aggressively cool them and hope they can ride it out. If they become refractory to all oxygenation therapies, the final therapy is ECMO. Sadly many patients are not candidates for ECMO due to a variety of appropriate reasons. There are many other reasons why patients may deteriorate, so we need to work quickly through a list of differential diagnoses. Thinking about the usual ICU culprits but also the nuances of COVID-19 infection. Whilst it is a devastating illness, it is also fascinating and unlike anything I have dealt with before.

Approximately a third of patients on the unit are doing well, gradually improving with a glimmer of hope that they will beat this *terrible disease and leave the ICU. Another third seem stuck. Still on mechanical ventilatory support. Still requiring kidney support and sometimes blood pressure support. And on a decent percentage of inspired oxygen. We can only hope that all these patients need is time. The final third are not doing well. On high amounts of organ support. Some on the maximum amount of oxygen we can deliver, but still they hold on. Everyone willing them to keep fighting and praying they turn the corner. It is a worrying time for us but utterly heartbreaking for the families. The only contact they get is daily updates via phone and online e-visiting via iPads.*

At around 11pm, I phone a patient's wife. He is relatively young, usually well, and has two young children. His wife is understandably incredibly anxious and has already phoned the unit a number of times tonight. My heart reaches out to her. I phone her, hoping to provide some comfort and reassurance. We chat for around 20 minutes. She is on her own having sent her children away to a relative. She can't eat or sleep. She is living a recurring nightmare. There is very little I can say to reassure her other than we won't give up on him. That we will continue to give our all to get him through this. He is one of the sickest patients on our unit. His body almost overwhelmed by the virus. But he is holding on. I can't give her false hope, but I can give her some hope. I tell her to try and rest. That I will call her if I am concerned. It is all I can do.

The rest of the night is spent troubleshooting ventilatory issues, tweaking medication, adjusting targets and ensuring each patient is stable for handover the next morning. I even manage a bit of teaching on ventilators for my junior colleagues, all bar two have been redeployed from other specialities and this is their first experience of ICU. Baptism of fire!

One patient who had a wobble at the start of the night seems to be significantly improving. Has he turned the corner this night? It looks like it and I feel emboldened. Hopefully one more to beat COVID-19.

And then its morning. We do a walk round handover with the day team. The 'Covid Tactical Commander' pops in for an update of events overnight. He looks pleasantly surprised at my reply to his question regarding how our night had been … 'it was a good night,' is my reply. He smiles wearily and says that it is refreshing to hear it. And it honestly was. All patients survived the night. Morale was good and our team provided excellent care under difficult circumstances. I feel proud of my department. And I feel hopeful for the NHS. Lockdown is working. The British public are behind us. Every time a new challenge arises, people step up.

But I am so aware that this is not the end. We have a long way to go and many challenges ahead. And whilst COVID-19 admissions decrease rapidly via ED and the wards, the ICUs will be busy with COVID-19 for a long time yet. Many patients continue to fight for their lives. There will be more losses. We must not forget those still fighting, their families or the staff caring for them.

20 April 2020

Early data suggests only 2-3 per cent of the population has been infected with COVID-19 according to WHO, meaning a large proportion of people remain susceptible. The number of people hospitalised with COVID-19 has begun to fall in Scotland, Wales and every region of England. Italy and Spain also report falls in their daily death tolls.

21 April 2020

The World Food Programme warns that the number of people suffering from acute hunger could surpass 250 million by the end of the year due to the pandemic. Deaths in England and Wales reach a twenty-year high according to figures released by the Office for National Statistics. The NHS Nightingale Hospital Yorkshire and the Humber is opened in Harrogate – Captain Tom Moore is the guest of honour. COVID-19 cases in Singapore surge with over 8,000 recorded infections. The country was praised for its efficient containment of the virus when it first emerged in February. The second wave is attributed to the migrant worker population who live in twenty-bed dormitories that make social distancing almost impossible.

My NHS Story

Dr Rebecca Daly is a UK trained GP, who was working in private practice in Singapore when the pandemic hit.

'I studied medicine at the University of Liverpool, where, in 1998, we were one of the first cohorts of students that utilised the problem-based learning approach. In conventional medical training, patient contact is deferred until the 3rd or 4th year, yet from day one we found ourselves fresh-faced, perched on hospital beds, poised to hear the patient's own narrative about their health care journey. As Williams Osler said: 'Listen to your patient, they are telling you the diagnosis.' Clinical contact was the core of our training and perhaps my future as a GP was being forged very early on.

After graduation, I rotated through several specialities within the NHS, and soon recognised my enjoyment of seeing the patient as a whole. I was left wanting to discover what happened next after discharge. I realised that general practice allowed me to provide holistic continuity of care to my patients, and inevitably I embarked on a GP training course at a busy practice in Westminster. Our community encompassed a wide demographic, and I relished seeing the whole of society walking through my door every day, from politicians and young families to heroin addicts and the homeless. There was never a dull day, as I worked within the hum of an inner-city area. This was the NHS at its best, free at the point of care, irrespective of nationality or income. Our services were constantly evolving and tailored to our practice population. We recruited a resident Bengali interpreter who became a pillar of support to our patients. We had an in-house community psychiatric nurse, which streamlined communication with our secondary care colleagues. The senior doctors were true family physicians, some of them serving their community for several decades, meaning they knew the needs of the patients well.

On completion of my training post, I strived to offer the same principles in my practice, to serve my patients in the NHS, getting to know them and their families, and contribute towards improving the delivery of care for our particular community. However, over time I recognised the frustration of rising bureaucracy that was impeding on the time available to truly listen to my patients. Government QOF targets meant the consultation would involve an interrogation of my patient on matters such as their smoking status, or whether their smear was due, often impeding the doctor–patient relationship. Meetings to discuss complex patients or coordinate palliative care were replaced by discussions of referral and prescribing targets in a complex game of ever-changing goalposts.

'The ongoing challenge to provide healthcare to a rising, aging population by successive governments has resulted in six national strategic plans since I started at medical school, all promising to improve the delivery of healthcare. Large scale reconfiguration of services have occurred at vertigo-inducing speed for most GPs, from Strategic Health Authorities, Primary Care Trusts, CCGs and more recently, the introduction of Sustainability and Transformation Plans.

'During my career, I have witnessed the first industrial action in over forty years as doctors protested against the NHS Pension scheme reforms in 2012. Later in 2016, it was the junior doctors calling a strike provoked by contractual changes proposed by government.

'During this same year, I found myself in my clinic room at 9pm staring bleary eyed at my computer screen, knowing my children were already in bed. I had not had a break since I started at 8am that morning, and I was still calling patients, much to their surprise. Over the years, the workload has increased in line with the demands upon the NHS, as austerity measures have taken their toll. Primary care was increasingly carrying the burden of secondary care, which was also buckling under the healthcare needs of the nation. I found myself supervising three paramedics, a nurse and a pharmacist, as allied healthcare professionals were increasingly utilised to lightened the load on GPs. This strategy only left us with more complex patients. The simple sore throat or bladder infection once served as a welcome opportunity to catch up on time during late running clinics. The 10-minute appointment had become outdated, in a world of escalating patient expectations, rising social needs unmet elsewhere, and the increasing complexity of primary care as we managed patients on long waiting lists.

'Referral criteria were tightened and increasingly scrutinised. Requests from patients to appeal secondary care decisions denying an operation soon added to the workload. Simultaneously, an era of rising litigation against doctors (despite evidence of improved healthcare delivery), and increasingly negative portrayal of doctors by the media was rapidly affecting morale. Despite all the extra work we were doing, there was less respect and support within the stretched system, causing doctors to leave in their droves, whilst the NHS staffing crisis deepened.

'I knew that something had to give and I decided to join the expanding number of Portfolio GPs. This new career path could provide more flexible working patterns to liberate oneself from the increasing burden of bureaucracy faced by permanent GPs. I pursued a locum career, and soon became the lead of the locum chambers of Kent and Sussex. I met a fantastic group of excellent GPs who treasured the day-to-day patient care but for diverse reasons had decided to turn their back on a conventional GP career. We held regular meetings and discussed interesting and complex cases, and I was struck by our collective enthusiasm for providing good patient care and our interest in medicine, yet at some point we had all become disillusioned with the traditional career path of the GP. I had not had similar enlightening meetings since early in my GP career, yet I relished this sharing of knowledge.

'Alongside this role, I worked in the local cottage hospital proving out-of-hours GP care. I set up contraceptive clinics for local GP practices and I also ventured into the emerging world of telemedicine, still providing NHS care but on a new modern platform. I had managed to forge a sustainable full-time career, whilst having a young family, and had acquired a more interesting, diverse scope of practice. The downside to this, however, was that my initial desire to serve the local community and provide holistic continuity of care had been sacrificed along the way. In 2019, I joined the increasing number of UK trained doctors turning their back on their beloved NHS and I moved with my family to Singapore to work as family doctor in an expat population.

'Suddenly, gone are the NHS standard blue walls, carpeted floors and long waiting times for appointments. I now work in the world of private medicine, where my patients are served cappuccinos and cookies in the waiting room. My prescribing practices and referral rates are not at the mercy of a local authority and I can facilitate a same-day specialist appointment for my patient with ease. Undeniably, the medicine is the same, however, I now have the time I need to sit with my patients and provide the holistic care all doctors strive for. I can deliver comprehensive preventative medicine, the backbone of primary care, being able to tailor health screening to the patient's risk factors rather than the national cost-effective programme. A new realisation dawned on me, that I had been rationing medicine my whole career, where budgets had often hampered clinical care, and treatment decisions were made based on cost per year of life saving.

Of course, private medicine can pose certain challenges too. I have had many difficult conversations with patients in the event their insurance will not cover their treatment. For instance, the domestic helper on minimum wage who is not able to afford basic screening tests and presents with late stage cervical cancer, such dilemmas unthinkable within the NHS. Without the rigorous recall system of the

NHS, patients can easily slip through the net, with the onus on the patient to attend important health checks. Private health care is more fragmented, whilst the coordination of care across the NHS facilitates doctors to collaborate and share knowledge with other allied health professionals such as social workers or health visitors, in a system where the vulnerable are not forgotten.

'On 3 January 2020, I was four months into my new job and still settling into our new life in Singapore when a circular from the Singaporean Ministry of Health landed on my desk. It warned of a cluster of cases of severe pneumonia of unknown cause in the city of Wuhan, China. A quick google of Wuhan and a mental note made of the particulars and I started my clinic, unaware that only twenty days later Singapore would see its first case, and even more unthinkable, that in two months' time the World Health Organisation would be announcing a global pandemic of what we now know as COVID-19. The management of this pandemic only highlighted the dichotomy between the health care systems of Singapore and the NHS.

'Singapore had a head start, as this was not the first pandemic suffered in recent years. Significant lessons had been learnt from the experience of SARS in 2003. Substantial pandemic preparation had occurred – a new National Centre of Infectious Disease had been built and contingency plans for managing PPE and food supplies in the state of a pandemic were drafted. People took it upon themselves to wear masks quite early on and temperature screening and disinfectant handwash were commonplace almost overnight. Within our own clinic, protocols were expedited as soon as the first case was announced in Singapore. To allow safe working practices, patients were screened for symptoms and travel history on the phone and at the clinic door. Patients and doctors undertook temperature screening twice a day. Anyone identified at high risk of COVID-19, were immediately referred for testing as Singapore initiated a rigorous test, isolate and trace policy.

'As I was being supplied with full PPE including gown, cap, goggles, FP3 mask and visor, I heard from colleagues back home about their struggles to find scrubs and of their ingenious ways of sourcing their own masks and goggles from hardware stores, or by relying on local school donations for protective goggles. I was even more aghast to hear of doctors being told they were not allowed to wear their own sourced PPE even though they were only provided with a surgical mask, apron and gloves for any face to face contacts.

'In this new COVID-19 world, Singapore's government was better placed to quickly implement measures to control the spread of a pandemic. Whilst I watched escalating statistics of loss of life in the UK after an earlier plan for herd immunity, Singapore was diligently wearing masks and logging all movements on a tracing app. Only a few days after the first case in Singapore, travel restrictions were implemented, with a two-week stay at home notice for returning Singaporeans. Non-adherence to the measures could result in a considerable fine, imprisonment or work visas for foreign nationals being revoked. A comprehensive policy commenced to test symptomatic patients, admit and isolate positive cases and then trace any potential contacts. This required considerable manpower, which came quite literally from an army of people, in the form of the National Servicemen of the Singapore Armed Forces.

When my son's teacher tested positive for COVID-19, I experienced the rigour of the Singapore test and trace system first hand. We were notified on the phone of the contact, and visited at the house by an officer from the Ministry of Health to serve our quarantine papers, dictating my son and a primary carer (myself) had to remain isolated in one room of the house until two weeks after the last contact with the positive case. We were supplied with a thermometer and were to expect video calls three times a day to confirm his temperature readings and to prove we were still isolating. We were warned of the possibility of random spot checks at the house and reminded of the disciplinary procedures for non-adherence. We were supplied with two surgical masks, to be used if we needed to travel to the hospital if he became symptomatic. We later received a card from the local community centre, encouraging us to call if we needed any help with groceries or other errands and to wish us good health.

'By 24th March, all short term visitors to Singapore were banned, even if transiting through the airport, and a trace app was in widespread use to help with tracking cases. During the same month in the UK, sporting events and other large-scale gatherings were still permitted. Pubs remained open with the onus on the public to not patronise them, and images of the Stereophonics playing to a crowd of 5,000 in Cardiff were being circulated around the world. The UK decided to adopt a mandatory two-week quarantine period for all travellers to the UK – but not until 22nd May. Flights had continued throughout this period, including from affected areas in China.

'Despite all this, watching from afar as the COVID-19 story unfolded in the UK, I have never felt so proud of the NHS and all it represents. Staff have shown an incredible ability to adapt and reorganise. I am aware of doctors volunteering to man 111 calls and provide their services to temporary hospitals, such as the Nightingale in London. I have seen primary and secondary care come together, sharing knowledge from their experience at the coal face of the pandemic. The ability to coordinate care on a large scale being demonstrated as doctors were deployed to other specialities and GPs rearranged clinics to be able to provide safe care to their patient communities. The NHS staff were holding up the health care of the country despite their lack of PPE, reaching out to those most vulnerable during these challenging times. My hopes for the future of the NHS is that we can learn from this pandemic. Primary care has had to question its delivery of services and consider what is achievable and necessary with limited resources. I am sure the telemedicine revolution will not subside with the end of COVID-19. I also hope the nation has a greater appreciation of the NHS with its finite resources, for it is an envied system that provides healthcare for all, free at the point of care.'

22 April 2020

Matt Hancock states in Commons that 'we are at the peak' of the pandemic, but social distancing measures cannot be relaxed. Professor Chris Whitty says the UK will have to live with some form of social distancing for at least the rest of the year.

23 April 2020

The first human trials of a COVID-19 vaccine in Europe begin in Oxford. Matt Hancock announces that all key workers and their household are eligible for COVID-19 tests, which can be booked through the government website and conducted at drive through centres (ninety-two across the country) or via home testing kits. Hancock also announces plans to restart contact tracing, by recruiting 18,000 staff to assist Public Health England.

24 April 2020

The UK COVID-19 testing website temporarily closes after high demand for the test.

25 April 2020
The number of recorded deaths in the UK reaches 20,319. Worldwide, this figure is 200,000. Figures show that ED attendances are half their usual level, raising concerns that people are putting off going to hospital due to COVID-19 fears.

26 April 2020
The benefits of social distancing are starting to be felt in the UK – 413 recorded deaths is the lowest daily total in April.

27 April 2020
The UK government announces that the families of healthcare workers who die due to COVID-19 will be entitled to a payment of £60,000. 360 deaths are recorded which is the lowest rise in four weeks. Australia begin to ease lockdown restrictions.

29 April 2020
Official figures in the UK start to include deaths in care homes and the community, meaning the number of recorded deaths increased by 4,419, to account for deaths occurring since 2nd March.

30 April 2020
Boris Johnson announces that the UK is 'past the peak' and that he will set out plans for easing lockdown next week.

1 May 2020
Donald Trump claims there is evidence that COVID-19 originated in a Chinese laboratory. Scientists have disproved this theory and the US have not provided the evidence they claim to have. Chinese state media called the claims 'insane'.

2 May 2020
£72 million of funding is to be made available to vulnerable people in the UK including victims of domestic violence and modern slavery who have suffered during the lockdown restrictions.

3 May 2020
An NHS Contact tracing app, aiming to limit a second wave, is trialled on the Isle of Wight. It relies on people downloading and using the app to be effective.

My NHS Story – Dr Jenny Abthorpe – Covid Diaries

4 May 2020

Today I went to work.

Sat on the train into London, watching the scenery rush past on a beautiful early Spring morning.

Pondering on the previous week's events when I had experienced a moment of real closure which had started a slow healing process for me.

I had been on-call for ED, the outward facing bleep for ICU. Not much was happening in ED in the early morning so I was assisting the Outreach team. I was delegated to go and review a patient who had stepped down from ICU. He had a tracheostomy and needed a review as to whether it could be removed. To my delight, it was the patient I had intubated on the ICU almost a month to the day. The one I had urged to 'do well'. It was one of those moments that is meant to be.

I arrived on his ward and went to say hello. As I approached his bed, I felt a rush of emotion. He looked fantastic! He looked quizzically at me but smiled with equal delight as I explained who I was. I told him that it meant a lot for me to see him. I delivered the good news that I felt it was the right time to remove his tracheostomy. He was understandingly nervous but after explanation and reassurance, I removed it.

Afterwards we chatted for a good while. He told me about his experience. His memories of his ICU stay (thankfully very little), his fears, his dreams for the future and his hope that he finally would make it home. He still refused to FaceTime or phone his son as he didn't want to get anyone's hopes up. But he had been texting. He said he would FaceTime the day he got home.

He was so grateful. We gave each other a hug. Both needing it as much as each other. And then I said goodbye and good luck. Leaving him in the care of his fantastic ward team. We had gone full circle and come out the other side.

Today it was business as usual. We have many patients doing well, some are a bit static but there are some truly miraculous recoveries. Patients that have defied all odds. We still have new admissions coming in with COVID-19 but these are low numbers and we feel we know our adversary better now. The expanded ICUs are being decompressed and cleaned. Redeployed staff are being moved back into their base specialties...hopefully inspired by their brief stint in ICU. I could never have predicted the incredible collaboration, teamwork and solidarity displayed by all specialties towards our ICU team. Long may it continue. We are so grateful to all of them. True heroes.

Now it's time to try and focus on our own recovery. As the pace slows, emotions start to surface. Images of lines of ventilated patients are not easily forgotten. Nor the countless breaking bad news phone-calls. Or patients reviewed and intubated in ED. Or the losses. But the healing has begun.

'My experience was mirrored up and down the UK, as the NHS reacted to an unprecedented challenge. The pandemic response by the NHS was immense and highly complex. A huge logistical challenge encompassing significant numbers of patients and their families, mobilising a large workforce, supplying vast amounts of PPE, medical equipment and drugs, rapidly expanding the number of ICU beds, training and educating redeployed staff and implementing national research trials at short notice. The NHS did not just cope, it saved thousands of lives. I will always be immensely proud of my profession and speciality in the part it played against COVID-19.'

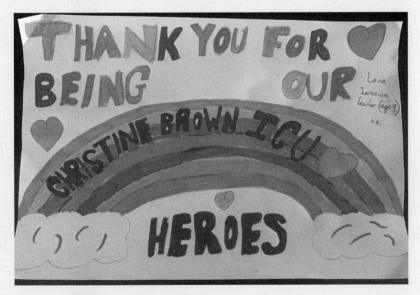

Thank you for being our NHS Heroes.

5 May 2020

The UK has the highest number of COVID-19 related deaths in Europe at 29,427. NHS Nightingale Hospital North East is opened near Sunderland by Health Secretary

Matt Hancock. Sir Patrick Vallance tells the House of Commons Health Select Committee that earlier testing for COVID-19 would have been beneficial, but would not have prevented the spread of the virus. WHO announce 108 potential COVID-19 vaccines in development around the world, with eight approved for clinical trials

7 May 2020

The government confirms that 400,000 gowns ordered from Turkey to increase PPE supplies have been impounded after failing to meet the required safety standards. Baroness Dido Harding, chair of NHS Improvement is appointed to lead the UK governments test and trace programme.

9 May 2020

UK Transport Secretary Grant Shapps announces £2 billion of investment to encourage walking and cycling, describing it as a 'once in a generation change' to the way the public travels.

10 May 2020

The UK government updates its COVID-19 message from 'stay at home, protect the NHS, save lives', to 'stay alert, control the virus, save lives'. Leaders of the devolved governments decide to stick with the original slogan. A new alert scale is announced ranging from level one (green-COVID-19 no longer present in the UK) to level five (red-COVID-19 epidemic is in general circulation and there is a risk of healthcare services being overwhelmed). The UKs plans to reopen society begins, with those who cannot work from home being encouraged to return to work the following day. Passengers arriving to the UK will be asked to quarantine for fourteen days from 8th June.

11 May 2020

People in the UK are advised by the government to wear face coverings on public transport and in shops. Teaching unions express concern at the government plan to reopen schools on 1st June.

12 May 2020
The UK's furlough scheme is extended until October. A quarter of the workforce, approximately 7.5 million people, are covered by the scheme, costing £14 billion a month

13 May 2020
The Health Protection (Coronavirus Restrictions) (England) (Amendment 2) Regulations 2020 come into effect allowing garden centres, sports courts and recycling centres to reopen. House moves and viewings are also permitted.

14 May 2020
NHS England compile a breakdown of underlying health conditions among those that died of COVID-19 in hospital between 31st March and 12th May. One in four had diabetes. Other common conditions include dementia (18 per cent), breathing problems (15 per cent), chronic kidney disease (14 per cent) and ischaemic heart disease (10 per cent). Public Health England approve a blood test that can detect COVID-19 antibodies.

15 May 2020
Matt Hancock announces that every resident and staff member in care homes throughout England will be tested for COVID-19 by early June.

16 May 2020
Spain and Italy plan to reopen some public places and Italy will lift travel restrictions from 3rd June, as the country records its lowest increased in COVID-19 deaths for two months

18 May 2020
Rail operators in the UK begin running more services. The London congestion charge is reinstated and buses begin charging passengers again. Jury trials resume. It is announced that anyone in the UK over the age of 5 with symptoms can now be tested for COVID-19. In Denmark, cafes, pubs and restaurants reopen.

19 May 2020
UK figures show there have been 11,600 deaths in care homes as a result of COVID-19. MPs are criticised for not prioritising care homes

earlier in the pandemic. Multiple security flaws are identified in the NHS COVID-19 tracing app and legislation is called for to prevent data being used for anything other than contact tracing. Global carbon emissions are at the lowest level in fifteen years.

20 May 2020
The number of people in hospital in the UK with COVID-19 drops below 10,000 for the first time since March. Boris Johnson promises that a track and trace system will be in place from 1st June. Cambridge University announces all lectures will be held online in the next academic year.

21 May 2020
A deal is agreed between the UK government and pharmaceutical company Roche to make a COVID-19 antibody test available through the NHS. Healthcare staff are the first to access it (this test checks to see if a person has had the virus. It cannot tell people if they are immune from catching COVID-19 again. The main value of this information at this point of the test is to build a picture of how many people have had the infection). The UK government announces that NHS staff will be exempt from the immigration health surcharge that is usually applied to non-EU migrants. Worldwide, the number of COVID-19 cases passes 5 million.

22 May 2020
The UK Scientific Advisory Group for Emergencies publishes its evidence on the safety of reopening schools from 1st June and declare the risk very, very small, but not zero.

23 May 2020
The UK Prime Minister's chief advisor Dominic Cummings comes under fire to resign after it is revealed he went against government guidance to drive 260 miles from London to Durham while his wife had symptoms of COVID-19. He later says in a press conference, 'I don't regret what I did', saying he needed to travel for childcare.

24 May 2020
Public Health England report that in samples from blood donors in London, antibodies indicating exposure to COVID-19 are present in around 16 per cent of people sampled. Boris Johnson confirms plans for a phased reopening of schools in England from 1st June.

27 May 2020
In New Zealand, hospitals have no more COVID-19 patients, and only twenty-one cases are reported in the country.

28 May 2020
Contact tracing systems are launched in England (NHS Test and Trace) and Scotland (Test and Protect). Baroness Dido Harding, head of the scheme, announces it will not be fully operational at a local level until the end of June.

29 May 2020
The COVID-19 technology access pool is launched by thirty countries and international partners as an initiative to share knowledge on vaccines, treatments and health technologies to fight COVID-19. NHS Seacole (named for British-Jamaican nurse Mary Seacole, a hero of the Crimean war) is opened in Surrey as a rehabilitation centre for COVID-19 patients who no longer need hospital care but cannot cope with their symptoms at home. Trump withdraws the US from WHO.

How did the NHS cope with COVID-19?

The UK's response to COVID-19 certainly has been 'World-beating' as Boris Johnson repeatedly told us it would be, but perhaps not in quite the way he envisioned. As we keep hearing, it is too early to evaluate how different countries have responded to the pandemic, since COVID-19 deaths are recorded in different ways around the world, and most mild cases of the disease are not tested, therefore not counted in the statistics.

However, the UK has surpassed the rest of Europe in the number of deaths reported, with 46,706[*] deaths at the time of writing. Per capita, this death toll is one of the highest in the world. How can the UK have fared so badly when it boasts a strong economy and infrastructure, world-leading scientists and an enviable health service?

An inquiry is inevitable, but a glance through the timeline of events earlier in this chapter shows the crisis unfolding. While other countries locked down rapidly, the UK's leader debated herd immunity and

---

[*] As we go to print, a review of how deaths from coronavirus are counted in England has reduced the UK death toll by over 5,000 to 41,329.

'taking it on the chin' on national TV. Large gatherings continued to take place and pubs remained open until 20th March. Advice from WHO was consistently ignored. Contact tracing was stopped in the UK early in the pandemic and WHO's 'test, test, test' mantra failed to be adopted until the outbreak had taken hold.

The staff of the NHS rose remarkably to the challenges posed by COVID-19, in spite of the dithering leadership of the government. Over the course of a few weeks, frontline staff adopted completely new ways of working to ensure both patients and staff could be protected. Hundreds of returning clinicians staffed NHS 111's CCAS, while General Practice moved entirely to telephone and video consulting, establishing local 'hot hubs' or 'red zone clinics', where patients with suspected COVID-19 could be assessed face to face. Paramedics donned PPE for all patient contacts, while Emergency Departments across the country modified their waiting rooms, cubicles and their triage processes to ensure any infection was contained and dealt with the sickest COVID-19 patients coming through their doors. Hospitals discharged those who were medically fit, to make room for the influx of patients, and Nightingale hospitals were built in anticipation of any overflow.

One of the biggest failings of the pandemic in the UK, has to be the woeful lack of personal protective equipment (PPE) available to NHS staff. In 2016, a pandemic simulation exercise (Exercise Cygnus) was carried out to demonstrate the effects of an influenza pandemic on the UK. It found that the UK was not ready to cope with a pandemic, revealing a shortage of critical care beds, ventilators and PPE. Then Health secretary Jeremy Hunt reportedly voted against stockpiling gowns and visors due to the expense. Staff raised concerns at the outset of the pandemic, reporting the shortages were putting them at risk. The DHSC confirmed in June that they had sourced and supplied a further 2 billion items of PPE to staff in England (numbers boosted by counting individual gloves rather than pairs). However, a BMA survey found that half of doctors working in high risk areas reported shortages of gowns and goggles, while many care homes reported paying inflated prices to source their own supplies. A recent BMJ study from China found that healthcare workers who were appropriately protected with PPE did not contract COVID-19 while working in highly exposed environments. China have reported the deaths of twenty-three healthcare workers. In the UK, more than 540 NHS staff and care workers have died during the pandemic.

Questions need to be answered for the families of the thousands of people who have died during the pandemic – whether due to COVID-19 itself, or due to other causes – triggered by the cessation of routine care. Did they died because they were frightened to go to hospital when they had their heart attack or stroke, because they didn't want to catch coronavirus? Did they died while waiting for their cancer surgery? Did they died because they were in a care home that was not adequately protected against the virus. The big question is could their death have been prevented? Was there more that could have been done?

It is essential to have a health system that functions during times of crisis and this pandemic has highlighted the cracks in our NHS. Our systems for communicable disease control have been slowly eroded and fragmented since the 1970s, when the role of Medical Officer for Health (MOH) was abolished. Historically, each locality employed a MOH, charged with public health responsibilities, with access to local public health laboratories. This steering role was replaced by community physicians and then centralised, and the laboratories transferred to NHS hospitals. In 2012, Public Health England (part of the NHS) was created to protect the public from disease, and local authorities (part of a different Government department) were given responsibility to run it – but with falling numbers of community control teams and fewer consultants in communicable disease control, serving 343 local authority areas in England from only nine regional hubs. It is no wonder we stopped contact tracing and testing so early in the pandemic – we did not have the resources, expertise or man power to do this. Our public health services need to be rebuilt with more involvement from experienced clinicians and more control for local teams to tailor their plans to their own communities, rather than being bound by generic centralised policies. At the end of August 2020, the Government announced that PHE is to be disbanded and reformed as a new agency.

The UK Government needs to rethink its plan. As this book goes to press, schools, pubs and restaurants have all reopened and cases are slowly on the rise as the second wave approaches. Let us hope lessons have been learned and we follow the example of countries like New Zealand and Australia in the management of further spikes.

"How the NHS coped with COVID-19" is due out in 2021. This book talks in more detail through the timeline of the pandemic, both in the UK and around the world. It addresses the issues faced by the NHS, examines the decisions made by those in power, and discusses what went wrong for the UK. Following the same format at this book, frontline workers offer their personal 'Covid Stories' and tell us their experiences of the pandemic

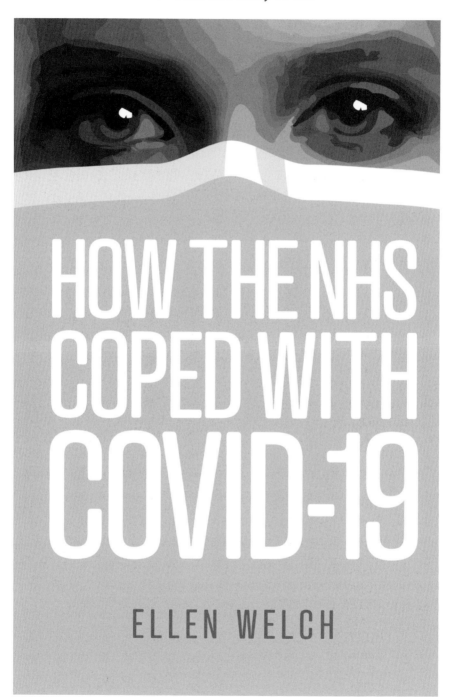

HOW THE NHS COPED WITH COVID-19

ELLEN WELCH

Sources and Additional Reading

Books and articles

ANDERSEN, K.G., RAMBAUT, A., LIPKIN, I., HOLMES, E.C., GARRY, R.F. (2020) The proximal origin of SARS-CoV-2. Nature Medicine 26: 450-452 https://www.nature.com/articles/s41591-020-0820-9

APPLEBY J, ABBASI K (2018) 'The NHS at 70: Loved, valued, affordable?' *BMJ* 361, 1540

BAIRSTOW, R. (2015) *The British Dentist*. Shire Library

BEGG N, RAMSAY M, WHITE J. (1998) 'Media dents confidence in MMR vaccine'. *BMJ 316, 561*

BEVAN, B., KARANIKOLOS,M., EXLEY, J., NOLTE, E., CONNOLLY, S. AND MAY, N. (2014) 'The four health systems of the United Kingdom: how do they compare?' Research report. The Nuffield Trust and Health Foundation

BREITNAUER, J. (2019) *The Spanish flu Epidemic and its influence on history*. Pen & Sword History

CARRIER E. (2013) 'High Physician Concern About Malpractice Risk Predicts More Aggressive Diagnostic Testing In Office Based Practice'. *Health Affairs* 32, 8, 383-1391

CRONIN, A.J. (1937) *The Citadel*. Pan Macmillan

DAVIS J, LISTER J, WRIGLEY D. (2015) *NHS for sale – Myths, lies and deception*. Merlin press.

DAVIS J, TALLIS R Ed. (2013) *NHS SOS - How the NHS was betrayed and how we can save it*. Oneworld

DAWSON, B. (1918) 'The future of the medical profession'. *Lancet*, 2, 83-85

DUCKWORTH, J. (2016) *Health and heartbreak - Healthcare before the NHS*. Austin Macauley Publishers Ltd

EL-GINGIHY Y (2015) *How to dismantle the NHS in 10 easy steps.* Zero Books

GODBER, G. (1988) 'Forty years of the NHS'. *BMJ*, 297, 37-43

GREEG, D. (2010) *Pauper Capital: London and the Poor Law 1790-1870.* Routledge, Aldershot

GRIST, N.R. (1979) *Pandemic Influenza* 1918. BMJ, 2: 1632-33 https://www.bmj.com/content/2/6205/1632

HONIGSBAUM, M. (2019) *The Pandemic Century: One Hundred Years of Panic, Hysteria, and Hubris.* C Hurst & Co Publishers Ltd.

HORTON, R. (2020) The COVID-19 Catastrophe. *What's gone wrong and how to stop it happening again.* Polity Press.

HUANG, C et al. (2020) Clinical features of patients infected with 2019 novel coronavirus in Wuhan, China. *The Lancet*, 395, 10223: 497-506 https://www.thelancet.com/journals/lancet/article/PIIS0140-6736(20)30183-5/fulltext

KMIETOWICZ, Z. (2006) *A century of general practice.* BMJ, 332, 7532, 39-40

LEWIS J, WILLIAMS A, FRANKLIN B, THOMAS J, MOSDELL N. (2008) *The Quality and Independence of British Journalism.* Cardiff: Cardiff University Media Department.

LIU, M., CHENG, SZ et al. (2020) Use of personal protective equipment against coronavirus disease 2019 by healthcare professionals in Wuhan, China: cross sectional study. BMJ; 369: 2195

LIU, S.L., SAIF, L.J., WEISS, S.R., SU, L. (2020) No credible evidence supporting claims of the laboratory engineering of SAR-CoV-2. Emerg. Microbes infect. 9: 505-507

MCCARTNEY M. (2016) *The state of medicine – keeping the promise of the NHS.* Pinter & Martin

MCDERMOTT I, CHECKLAND K et al (2016) 'Engaging GPs in commissioning: realist evaluation of the early experiences of Clinical Commissioning Groups in the English NHS'. J Health Serv Res Policy, 22, 1, 4–11.

NASH L.M. (2010) 'Perceived practice change in Australian doctors as a result of medicolegal concerns'. *MJA* 193, 579-583

NIGHTINGALE, F. (1898) *Notes on Nursing What it is and What it is not.* D Appleton and Company, New York

PARKES, M & SHEARD, S. (2012) *Nursing in Liverpool since 1862.* Scotforth Books, Lancaster

PARKIN, E. (2020) The prescription charge and other NHS charges. House of Commons Library. Briefing Paper number 07227

PINDER, RJ. (2014) *The NHS in England An introduction for junior doctors.* Codex Project, London

POLLOCK, A., RODERICK, P., CHENG, K.K. (2020) COVID-19: why is the UK government ignoring WHO's advice? BMJ, 368:1284

POLLOCK, AM (2005) NHS Plc: *The Privatisation of our health care*. Verso Books

POLLOCK, AM (2016) *The End of the NHS*. Verso Books

RICHARDSON, R. (2013) 'A dismal prospect: Workhouse Healthcare'. *Lancet*, 382, 20-21

RIVETT, G. (1998) *From Cradle to Grave: Fifty years of the NHS*. King's Fund, London

RIVETT, GC (1986) *The development of the London hospital system 1823-1982*. London, King's Fund

ROBERTS, F. (1949) 'The cost of the NHS'. *BMJ*, 1, 293

ROGERS, J. (1889) *Reminiscences of a workhouse medical officer*. Fisher Unwin, London

SMITH, H.L. (2014) *Harry's last stand*. Icon Books Ltd

SPINNEY, L. (2017) *Pale Rider: The Spanish flu of 1918 and How it changed the World*. Vintage

STUDDERT DM. (2005) 'Defensive Medicine Among High Risk Specialist Physicians in a Volatile Malpractice Environment'. *JAMA* 293, 21, 2609-2617

TAYLOR R. (2013) *God Bless the NHS-The truth behind the current crisis*. Faber & Faber guardianbooks

VAN BEKKUM JE, HILTON S. (2013) 'Primary care nurses' experiences of how the mass media influence frontline healthcare in the UK'. *BMC Fam Pract* 14, 178

WATSON, R. (1969) *Edwin Chadwick, Poor Law and Public Health*. Longman, Essex

WHITBY, L. (1948) 'The Changing Face of Medicine'. *BMJ*, 4565, 2-6

WHITFIELD, M. (2016) *The Dispensaries. Healthcare for the poor before the NHS. Britains forgotten health-care system*. AuthorHouse UK, Bloomington, USA

WILSON, N., GELBIER, S. (2014) *The Changes in Dentistry since 1948: The John McLean Archive – A Living History of Dentistry Witness Seminar 2*. British Dental Association

WOOLHANDLER S, HIMMELSTEIN DU (1997) 'Costs of care and administration at For-Profit and other hospitals in the United States'. *NEJM* 336, 769-774

Online sources

AMNESTY INTERNATIONAL UK. UK among highest COVID-19 health worker deaths in the world. 13 Jul 2020. https://www.amnesty.org.uk/press-releases/uk-among-highest-covid-19-health-worker-deaths-world

APPLEBY, J (2018) '70 years of NHS spending'. Nuffield Trust https://www.nuffieldtrust.org.uk/news-item/70-years-of-nhs-spending

Beveridge, W. (1942) Social Insurance and Allied Services (The Beveridge Report) available:

BMA (2018) Career break advice for GPs. https://www.bma.org.uk/advice/career/progress-your-career/career-break-gp-advice

CARR, H (2018) Why is there always a winter crisis in the NHS? Sky News https://news.sky.com/story/why-is-there-always-a-winter-crisis-in-the-nhs-11195502

CENTRES FOR DISEASE CONTROL AND PREVENTION (2020) Public Health Responses to COVID-19 Outbreaks on Cruise Ships – Worldwide, February-March 2020. https://www.cdc.gov/mmwr/volumes/69/wr/mm6912e3.htm#F1_down

The COVID-19 technology access pool (C-TAP) https://www.who.int/emergencies/diseases/novel-coronavirus-2019/global-research-on-novel-coronavirus-2019-ncov/COVID-19-technology-access-pool

DAVIES, M (2018) GP dilemma: A patient from overseas expects me to prescribe antibiotics. https://www.gponline.com/gp-dilemma-patient-overseas-expects-prescribe-antibiotics/article/1461364

DAYAN, M., WARD, D., GARDNER, T., KELLY, E. (2018) How good is the NHS? https://www.kingsfund.org.uk/publications/nhs-70-how-good-is-the-nhs

Dentaid Charity website https://www.dentaid.org/uk/

DEPARTMENT OF HEALTH AND SOCIAL CARE (2019) DHSC's agencies and partner organisations https://www.gov.uk/government/publications/how-to-contact-department-of-health-arms-length-bodies/department-of-healths-agencies-and-partner-organisations

Department of Health. (2015) The NHS Constitution. Williams Lee. Available here: https://www.gov.uk/government/publications/the-nhs-constitution-for-england (

Florence Nightingale museum website. http://www.florence-nightingale.co.uk

GMC https://www.gmc-uk.org

GP Induction and Refresher Scheme. GP National recruitment office. https://gprecruitment.hee.nhs.uk/induction-refresher

HOLMES F. (2020) COVID-19 Timeline. British Foreign Policy Group. https://bfpg.co.uk/2020/04/COVID-19-timeline/

https://sourcebooks.fordham.edu/halsall/mod/1942beveridge.asp

https://www.bda.org/news-centre/press-releases/Pages/NHS-charges-masking-cuts-and-driving-patients-to-GPs.aspx

HUME R. (2020) 'Far too little too late' what happened when Spanish flu hit Britain a century ago. https://www.historyextra.com/period/first-world-war/spanish-flu-britain-how-many-died-quarantine-corona-virus-deaths-pandemic/

Kings Fund (2017) How the NHS is funded https://www.kingsfund.org.uk/projects/nhs-in-a-nutshell/how-nhs-funded

LAUER SA., GRANTZ MS et al (2020) The Incubation period of coronavirus disease 2019 (COVID-19) From publicly reported confirmed cases: estimation and application. Annals of Internal Medicine https://annals.org/aim/fullarticle/2762808/incubation-period-coronavirus-disease-2019-COVID-19-from-publicly-reported

MATTHEWS-KING A. (2015) Hunt confirms rollback on pre-election pledge of 5000 new GPs. Pulse. http://www.pulsetoday.co.uk/news/new-deal-2015/16/hunt- confirms-rollback-on-pre-election-pledge-of-5000-new-gps/20010348.fullarticle

MILLETT D. (2016) MPs Slam government 'complacency' over GP workforce crisis. GP Online. http://www.gponline.com/mps-slam-government-complacency-gp- workforce-crisis/article/1386541

Ministry of Health and Department of Health for Scotland. (1944) A National Health Service. London, HMSO. http://old.post-gazette.com/pg/pdf/201004/2010_national-health-service-book_01.pdf

MORAN V, ALLEN P et al. (2017) How are clinical commissioning groups managing conflicts of interest under primary care co-commissioning in England? A qualitative analysis http://bmjopen.bmj.com/content/7/11/e018422

MURPHY S (2018) NHS crisis? What crisis? http://www.dailymail.co.uk/news/article-5320623/NHS-doctors-ski-break-winter-emergency.html

National Health Service History http://www.nhshistory.net/

National life tables, UK: 2014-2016. (2017) Office for National Statistics. https://www.ons.gov.uk/peoplepopulationandcommunity/birthsdeathsandmarriages/lifeexpectancies/bulletins/nationallifetablesunitedkingdom/2014to2016

National Union of Journalists. (2011) NUJ Code of Conduct. Available: https://www.nuj.org.uk/about/nuj-code/

NAVARRO V (2003) 'The inhuman state of US Healthcare'. *Monthly Review*, 55, 4 https://monthlyreview.org/2003/09/01/the-inhuman-state-of-u-s-health-care

NHS Workforce Statistics, September 2017, Provisional Statistics https://digital.nhs.uk/catalogue/PUB30165

OCED. (2017) Health at a Glance 2017: OCED Indicators. OCED Publishing, Paris http://dx.doi.org/10.1787/health_glance-2017-en

Performer list policies and procedures. NHS England. https://www.england.nhs.uk/commissioning/primary-care/primary-care-comm/performer-list-policies-procedures/

REUTERS NEWS AGENCY. 11 Jan 2020. China reports first death from mysterious outbreak in Wuhan. Aljazeera https://www.aljazeera.com/news/2020/01/china-reports-death-mysterious-outbreak-wuhan-200111023325546.html

205

REUTERS NEWS AGENCY. 15 May 2020. Timeline: UK government advice on restricting visits to care homes https://www.reuters.com/article/us-health-coronavirus-britain-carehomes-idUSKBN22R2F0

ROBERTSON R., EWBANK L. (2020) Thinking differently about commissioning. The King's Fund https://www.kingsfund.org.uk/sites/default/files/2020-02/TBAC%20report%20%28web%29.pdf

RUSSELL P. (2020) Covid 19: Timeline of a pandemic. Medscape. https://www.medscape.com/viewarticle/927474

SPINNEY L. (2017) How the 1918 Flu Pandemic revolutionised public health https://www.smithsonianmag.com/history/how-1918-flu-pandemic-revolutionized-public-health-180965025/

TATTERSFIELD H (2013) GPs are already wise to the scam of new commissioning groups. The *Guardian* https://www.theguardian.com/commentisfree/2013/jan/21/gps-sham-ccgs-local-commissioning

Vaccinations – In 1948, children would be given smallpox and diphtheria vaccinations routinely. Today, the routine immunization schedule protects against 17 diseases (see here: https://www.gov.uk/government/uploads/system/uploads/attachment_data/file/633693/Complete_imm_schedule_2017.pdf for an up to date version of the routine immunization schedule

VAID N. (2010) 'Private sector providers in England: The implications of Independent sector treatment centres'. *Eurohealth*, 16, 3, 8-11 http://www.euro.who.int/__data/assets/pdf_file/0007/129436/Eurohealth16_3.pdf

WHO Best Practices for the naming of new human infectious diseases (Geneva: World Health Organisation, May 2015) https://apps.who.int/iris/bitstream/handle/10665/163636/WHO_HSE_FOS_15.1_eng.pdf;jsessionid=E693B4FE32A5F6593C46BCF0FFEEDFCC?sequence=1

WHO Timeline – COVID-19 https://www.who.int/news-room/detail/27-04-2020-who-timeline---COVID-19

WILLIAMS H, LEES C, BOYD M. (2014) the General Medical Council: fit to practice? Civitas Doctors Policy Research Group http://www.civitas.org.uk/pdf/GMCFittoPractise.pdf

Workhouses website. http://www.workhouses.org.uk

ZHAN, M. et al. (2020) Death from COVID-19 of 23 healthcare workers in China. NEJM 382; 2267-2268

Index